SEX GUIDE FOR COUPLES

Improve your sex life and have great sex, knowing what men and women really want. Explore your fantasies and have more intimacy for an amazing relationship. Play, gadget, sex toy

DONNA DARE

© **Copyright 2019 - All rights reserved.**

The content contained within this book may not be reproduced, duplicated or transmitted without direct written permission from the author or the publisher.
Under no circumstances will any blame or legal responsibility be held against the publisher, or author, for any damages, reparation, or monetary loss due to the information contained within this book. Either directly or indirectly.

Legal Notice:
This book is copyright protected. This book is only for personal use. You cannot amend, distribute, sell, use, quote or paraphrase any part, or the content within this book, without the consent of the author or publisher.

Disclaimer Notice:
Please note the information contained within this document is for educational and entertainment purposes only. All effort has been executed to present accurate, up to date, and reliable, complete information. No warranties of any kind are declared or implied. Readers acknowledge that the author is not engaging in the rendering of legal, financial, medical or professional advice. The content within this book has been derived from various sources. Please consult a licensed professional before attempting any techniques outlined in this book.
By reading this document, the reader agrees that under no circumstances is the author responsible for any losses, direct or indirect, which are incurred as a result of the use of information contained within this document, including, but not limited to, — errors, omissions, or inaccuracies.

Table of Contents

DESCRIPTION 1
INTRODUCTION 5
CHAPTER 1: COMMUNICATION 12
    LISTENING EFFECTIVELY 12
    I AND ME 13
    LEAVE THE PAST WHERE IT IS! 13
    DON'T ASSUME – ASK 14
    ACKNOWLEDGE AND RESPOND 14
    TONE OF VOICE 15
    YOU'RE NOT AT WORK NOW 15
    TAKING A TIME-OUT 16
    RESPECT YOUR PARTNER 16
CHAPTER 2: WHEN YOUR SPOUSE ISN'T INTERESTED IN SEX: COMMUNICATING YOUR NEEDS 18
CHAPTER 3: THE MALE AND FEMALE PSYCHE 26
CHAPTER 4: SEXLESS MARRIAGE 30
    REMOVE EMOTIONAL DISTANCES: 31
    ADMIRE EACH OTHER: 32
    MAKE YOUR FIGURE APPEALING: 32
    MAKE SURE TO HAVE SAFE ENVIRONMENT: 33
    PRIORITIZE INTIMACY: 34
    OPEN THE PATHS OF COMMUNICATION: 34
    EXTENDS THE WAYS FOR JOY ABLE ORGASM: 35

ADD MUSIC: 35

CHAPTER 5: EVERYBODY'S DIFFERENT 37
    Physical types 38
    Levels of passion (libido) 40

CHAPTER 6: HOW TO FALL BACK IN LOVE WITH YOUR PARTNER.. 45

CHAPTER 7: TALK DIRTY TO ME 50

CHAPTER 8: HOW TO SPICE THINGS UP IN THE BEDROOM... 55
    WEAR RED 55
    YOGA 55
    BE VOCAL 56
    COMEDY 56
    MORNING SEX 56
    EXERCISE 57
    PURPLE 57
    WINE 58
    MEN SHOULD DRINK, TOO.......................................58
    TRY SOMETHING NEW 58

CHAPTER 9: PREPARE YOUR TEMPLE OF LOVE; YOUR BODY 60
    BUILDING LOVE FOR YOUR BODY THROUGH THE LOOKING GLASS..60
    THE CONNECTION BETWEEN YOGA AND TANTRIC SEX 62
    Simple yoga movements.....................................62
    The head lift. 62

The cobra – pose. 63

The cat – pose. 63

The resting – pose. 63

THE FOOD YOU EAT IS WHAT DEFINES YOU 64

CHAPTER 10: HOW TO REACH YOUR MAXIMUM PLEASURE 65

INCREASING THE ODDS OF ORGASM IN WOMEN 65

POSITIONS THAT SATISFY BOTH PARTNERS....................... 68

CHAPTER 11: SEX AND PARTNER BONDING 70

A LASTING AFTERGLOW 71

A METAPHOR FOR INTIMACY 72

HAVE MORE SEX 73

CHAPTER 12: STAGES OF SEXUAL AROUSAL IN HUMANS 77

THE SENSUAL TOUCH 77

THE TEASING LICK 78

THE LICK BLOW 78

THE ORAL FLICK 79

THE ONE-TWO COMBO 79

THE SUCK AND SEAL 79

THE ORAL FINGER COMBO 80

THE SLOW THRUST.. 80

THE MISSIONARY DIVE 81

THE PILLOW BOOST 81

THE G-SPOT PUSH 82

The Head Rush 82

The Rocking Chair Thrust 83

CHAPTER 13: WAYS TO MAKE YOU LAST LONGER IN BED 84

CHAPTER 14: PREMATURE EJACULATION 94

CHAPTER 15: HOW TO RE-LIGHT THE SPARK – 15 WAYS TO FALL BACK IN LOVE 100

CHAPTER 16: SEXUAL ROLE-PLAYING GAMES 109

CHAPTER 17: SETTING THE MOOD 114

CHAPTER 18: OVERCOMING SEXUAL INHIBITIONS 120

CHAPTER 19: CRAZY POSITIONS AND PLACES/SITUATION WHERE TO HAVE SEX (EX WASHING MACHINE, ON THE STAIRS, ETC) SPICY TIPS 125

CHAPTER 20: SECRET TO LASTING LONGER 138

CHAPTER 21: ADVENTUROUS POSITIONS 148

CHAPTER 22: ADDITIONAL TIPS FOR BETTER SEX . 156

CONCLUSION 160

Description

So, you want to keep things spicy and fun in your relationship? Good! Now, let's get it done! There's a difference between wanting to do something and actually following through with it. Many relationships fail because what they want is much different than what they actually follow through with. Sexy lingerie, dirty talk and dirty text messages are all great ways to spice up any relationship. If you find that these areas aren't providing enough satisfaction, try something new. When you're in a relationship and you feel comfortable with someone, you must be willing to try new things. This doesn't necessarily mean that you have to try things that you're not comfortable with, but it does however mean that you should try things at least once (unless you're super uncomfortable with them or they are dangerous) and expand your way of thinking! Trying something new may involve dressing up for your partner. Now, yes, sexy lingerie is great and works wonders but this too can get boring and you then have to try new things! Start the discussion with your partner and find out what their fantasies are. Your woman may tell you that she's always dreamt of having a sexy police officer handcuff her and dive deep inside of her and your man may express to you that he wants to be whipped by cat woman. Whatever their fantasies are, do whatever you can to please them and fulfill their fantasies.

Take a trip to the local sex shop. Take a look around together. This is a great way to see what they offer at these stores and you can see what you're actually interested in. Your woman may decide that she wants you to use a vibrator on her and when she's there she can either pick it out, or just point out what she wants, that way you can go back later and surprise her with it.

Don't let the need for other items being brought into the bedroom make you feel as though you aren't doing enough. Adding items into the bedroom makes the experience more erotic and will provide for a great deal of pleasure for both individuals. For example, if you're bending your woman over and she needs her clitoris stimulated, try using a small vibrator on her. While you're penetrating her, you can reach your hand underneath and rub her clitoris with it while you're deep inside of her. This will really encourage an orgasm and you'll be able to see how she responds to this type of sexual activity. You also may be able to pleasure your man more by purchasing different types of lubricant that will allow him to go deeper inside of you.

This guide will focus on the following:

- Communication
- When your spouse isn't interested in sex: communicating your needs
- The male and female psyche
- Sexless marriage
- Everybody's different
- How to fall back in love with your partner
- Talk dirty to me
- How to spice things up in the bedroom
- Prepare your temple of love; your body
- How to reach your maximum pleasure
- Sex and partner bonding
- Stages of sexual arousal in humans
- Ways to make you last longer in bed
- Premature ejaculation
- How to re-light the spark – 15 ways to fall back in love
- Sexual role-playing games
- Setting the mood
- Overcoming sexual inhibitions

- Crazy positions and places/situation where to have sex (ex washing machine, on the stairs, etc) spicy tips
- Secret to lasting longer
- Adventurous positions
- Additional tips for better sex... AND MORE!!!

There are a million different items that you can incorporate into the bedroom. You just have to find what feels the best and what works for you and your relationship. Be open to new things and explore different areas. You never know where you will find pleasure!

Introduction

A few individuals think sex is misrepresented in a relationship. When you are enamored, it can join you two in a way dissimilar to whatever other. Besides the conspicuous interfacing part to having that time with your spouse, there are some extraordinary health advantages too. Reasons why sex is critical are all underneath, in spite of the fact that there are numerous more I'm certain.

Connects you

This is a standout amongst the most clear reasons why sex is critical I think. Obviously getting physically involved with each other is going to bring both of you closer. The basic truth that you are seeing one another stripped is sufficient to bring you closer. Once in a while being all that much enamored and being pulled in to one another, doesn't mean the sexual science arrives. When both of you have discovered your furrow in the room, you ought to see that science meeting up.

Stress release

That is to say, who wouldn't like to return home following a long distressing day and discharge that with some uproarious Os? This is an awesome approach to put another jump in your stride and restore your vitality, and obviously to disregard your taxing day. Specialists say individuals who have customary sex react preferable to stretch over people who don't.

Live longer

Having one climax a day can keep the specialist away (see what I did there?). All together for the ideal medical advantages, having a climax like clockwork keeps the wellbeing benefits at their greatest and the levels of oxytocin, estrogen and testosterone reliably streaming. That as well as standard sex can enhance cardiovascular wellbeing, diminish the dangers of prostate growth and even lessen the likelihood of osteoporosis. Why not help your spouse live more?

Exercise

Make your hot time into an activity! You really blaze 144+ calories for each half-hour each time you take care of business as per studies, and who doesn't love smoldering calories? (Particularly while having hot time!) The key for fatty blazing sex is making it hot and making it last, say specialists. You can likewise include a touch of groaning and murmuring, which can offer you some assistance with burning an additional 18 to 30 calories.

Good night's sleep

Who isn't drained after some time between the sheets? This is a fabulous approach to help you close those overwhelming eyes before your typical time. Sex is said to bring about a drop in body temperature, furthermore seems to incite a profound rest. Specialists, as a rule, debilitate exercise inside of a couple of hours of sleep time however the physical act of sex is by all accounts a positive exemption to that run the show.

Self-esteem

In the event that you are having intercourse with your spouse, you feel awesome about yourself, correct? In the event that you aren't, you ponder where else he is getting it. Having that time together demonstrates one another that you are conferred and you are enamored with one another. Presently obviously, in the event that you aren't engaging in sexual relations yet with your spouse, that is fine! Having some quality lip locking time does the trap generally too.

Keeps things hot

Sex is an awesome approach to revive by the day's end and to separate your schedule. On the off chance that you do the standard schedule each day, take a stab at tossing in hot time haphazardly. This will keep your relationship hot and unconstrained. What guy doesn't love that? You will as well!

Improves bladder control

You won't have issues holding your bladder now, but rather it's certain to happen later on. Then again, on the off chance that you have intercourse regularly enough, your bladder control will progress. It's most likely not your principal purpose behind engaging in sexual relations, but rather it's surely an awesome advantage!

Boosts libido

The more you engage in sexual relations, the more you'll need to have intercourse. So regardless of the fact that you're somewhat risky on intercourse now, you'll wind up being as energetic as a little bunny rabbit. The same will happen with your spouse, so both of you won't have any desire to keep your hands off of one another.

Glowing skin

Don't you cherish looking in the mirror to see faultless skin? All things considered, you'll be most of the way there once you begin engaging in sexual relations as often as possible. The more you do it, the better your skin will look. You'll have a sure gleam to you that isn't just because of your bliss.

Relieves pain

Having a cerebral pain is a repulsive reason for skipping out on sex. Why? Since sex can really cure a headache. It makes the agony vanish, so in case you're not feeling the best, engaging in sexual relations could be a decent move.

Fun

Why might you prevent yourself from accomplishing something fun? When you're with the right individual, you'll cherish each second you go through with them- - particularly the time you spend bare. A relationship is intended to make you more content, so all the fun is a piece of a vocation.

Easier to relax or breathe

Sex is "a characteristic antihistamine, combatting feed fever and asthma indications." That implies that it makes it simpler for you to relax. So on the off chance that you've been having issues with your sensitivities recently, a great come in the feed could be the cure you've been searching for.

Feeling of well-being

Engaging in sexual relations often will make a sentiment prosperity, which is the reason you nod off so effectively in the wake of doing it. That implies that intercourse helps both your body and your psyche. There's nothing undesirable about it.

Strengthens cardiac muscles

Sex isn't useful for your heart as far as your enthusiastic state. It's likewise useful for your physical wellbeing. On the off chance that you need your heart to stay solid, sex is an extraordinary approach to ensure that your blood continues pumping.

Intelligence

Sex can possibly support your knowledge. There are studies that demonstrate that it can "quicken cerebrum cell development." So in case you're wanting to pro a test, you can enjoy a reprieve from concentrating on to have some sex. Hey, it's justified regardless of a shot, would it say it isn't?

Stops boredom

When you go through huge amounts of time with your beau, things can get exhausting. When you come up short on things to do, sex is dependably an extraordinary movement to fall back on. Its something that'll never get stale, in light of the fact that there will dependably be a lot of new moves to experiment with.

Helps you know one another

You need your partner to know you all around. That implies that he ought to figure out how to joy you. The all the more regularly you engage in sexual relations, the better he'll get at making you upbeat. That is the reason you ought to peel off your garments at whatever point you can.

You'll look much younger

Everything on this rundown consolidated will help you look more youthful. At this moment, you won't not be agonized over wrinkles, but rather you will be later on. That is the reason having as much sex as you can while you can is an extraordinary thought.

I think we all know sex is essential in a relationship, obviously, on the off chance that you aren't at that stage yet, don't take this article the wrong way. Be that as it may, on the off chance that you are, then the above tips are all genuine, and trust, I am talking from my experience.

Chapter 1: Communication

The biggest issue facing all relationships at one point or another is communication. It's not just about not talking to each other; it's also about HOW you talk to each other. There are a number of common mistakes couples make when communicating, including not listening to what the other has to say. Many people make the mistake of reacting rather than responding to something that is said, and these reactions often are things said in the heat of the moment. Unfortunately, it is these comments that can do the most damage. Learning how to communicate effectively can help you keep your marriage or relationship on track.

Listening Effectively

During an argument, they often escalate because one or more of the parties doesn't feel as though they are really being listened to. You can hear something being said, but you are not always listening to what it is they are trying to convey to you. It becomes a back and forth situation, with each person waiting to have their say, and while they are waiting they are considering what they are going to say next rather than listen to what their partner is saying.

When your partner is talking to you, stop what you are doing and pay attention. Don't look at your phone, or walk into the next room. Stop physically doing anything and look at your partner while they are speaking. When they feel they have your undivided attention, they will think they are being heard. Wait until he or she has stopped talking before you respond – don't interrupt and this will show you are listening.

I and Me

Two words you should use when talking about how you feel about something, are I and Me. If you need your partner to do something in particular, explain why, and by using I or me, you will demonstrate how it is making you feel if they don't do it. By making it about what you need or feel, your partner won't feel as though they are being attacked. This will lead to more positive communication.

Leave the Past Where It Is!

Many of us are guilty of dragging up something from the past, particularly during an argument. You may be discussing or disagreeing about something that is present day, then all of a sudden bring up something that happened years ago that you felt was a slight towards you. All this does is make the argument escalate, as you are now not only arguing about a current issue, but also something that occurred ages ago. Thus, you have created 2 arguments in one! If your partner did something they shouldn't have a long time ago, and you obviously forgave them for it or you wouldn't still be with them, then don't drag it out every time you get into a heated discussion. The past is the past and that's where it should stay.

Don't Assume – Ask

If you don't understand something your partner has said, don't just assume you know. You need to ask them to explain, especially if your partner seems upset about the issue. Jumping to conclusions and making assumptions can lead to all sorts of communication issues between partners.

Acknowledge and Respond

Here is another good example of when the use of the word 'I' can be important. First listen to what your partner has to say, and then take a pause for a moment. This is the acknowledgement. Then, respond by using I, for example, 'I can see that you are not happy about....'. This shows that you are recognizing the feelings of your partner. Then, if necessary, explain to your partner why they may have the facts wrong, but do so in a calm manner. What you have succeeded in doing, is listening to what they have to say, acknowledged it, shown that you can see how they feel, then responded.

Tone of Voice

You have probably heard others say that it is not what is said, but how it is said that can make the big difference when communicating. This is absolutely true. You need to keep your voice at a calm level, not loud and shouting. You also need to make sure there is no hint of sarcasm or derision in your voice when you speak to your loved one.

You're Not At Work Now

Often partners make the mistake of arguing with their significant other just as they would with a work colleague. At work you may speak with a sterner tone, or you may use bullet points and facts to prove your point. When having a discussion with your partner however, you need to remind yourself that they have feelings and thoughts and if you treat them disrespectfully or harshly as you might a co-worker, this can make them feel vulnerable. Don't bully your partner, or make them feel as though they are beneath you in any way, shape or form.

Taking a Time-Out

If you are engaging in a discussion with your partner and it is heating up to a full-blown shouting argument, call a time-out. This enables you both to calm down and think rationally, before all the unnecessary remarks and accusations can occur. Agree to continue the discussion later, once the situation has cooled. This allows both of you to gather your thoughts and focus on the issue at hand rather than dragging up everything else at the same time.

Respect Your Partner

The greatest thing you can show your partner is respect. Always treat them how you would like to be treated. They are not below you, they are your equal, and making them feel any less than that will destroy your relationship. This includes when you are out socially, as how you make your partner feel when out with other people will determine how they feel about you. If you put him or her down in front of others, it will result in a great deal of damage between you.

Chapter 2: When Your Spouse Isn't Interested In Sex: Communicating Your Needs

Get Your Heart Right

Try not to enter a discussion furious or intense. On the off chance that your life partner has wronged you, go to God with that outrage and request that he offer you some assistance with forgiving. You need a discussion where you seek what is best for you as a couple. Having a discussion where you're attempting to get him or her to recognize the amount they've harmed you won't as a matter, of course, help your relationship. There is a period to bring this up, once things are looking better, yet in the event that the longing is to move your relationship towards more noteworthy closeness, that is the thing that you ought to be concentrating on, not retaliation. God calls us to adore our life partners wholeheartedly, regardless of the possibility that they don't address our issues.

Concentrate on Closeness, not Sexual Discharge

Your life partner has an issue with sex. Odds are they discover it a fairly distasteful–if not extremely distasteful–obligation. It could be on account of they have truly negative demeanors about sex, or it could just be on account of they're drained, they're tired of having things on their schedule, and they would prefer not to need to accomplish something vivacious that they need to "get in the mind-set" for.

On the off chance that you discuss your sexual needs, odds are this is the thing that your companion will listen: "I have sexual needs in light of the fact that I have never truly created restraint the way you have.

I am a slave to my body, not at all like you, why should capable spotlight on the critical things in life. What's more, now, as a result of my yearning and absence of discretion, I need you, who are as of now occupied, to get lively and to imagine that you really need sex with the goal that I can get some discharge."

Not precisely an extremely appealing recommendation, is it? Clearly, that is not what you mean, but rather regardless of the fact that you essentially said something like this: I fancy you. I discover you so appealing. You energize me. I need us to encounter this together. I need to feel adored.

Your life partner will hear the first piece, particularly if this has turned into a major zone of contention in your relationship.

So what would it be advisable for you to do? Concentrate on the genuine issue–the one that both of you share. You need more closeness, and sex is an entryway into closeness. I would say something like this:

I truly trust that God made us to yearn for one another and to have the capacity to encounter significant profundities of adoration and closeness. I trust that God needs us to feel energetic about one another, near one another, and really imply, with the goal that we realize that we're definitely not strolling through life alone. I need us to feel so frantically infatuated, and I need you to feel the amount I cherish you. I need us to feel like we're absolutely one, and I trust that the way that God made us to express that is through sex.

I know sex can be troublesome for you, and I know you're drained a great deal of the time. I know you have an inclination that you don't have a ton of longing. Yet, I'm concerned that our absence of closeness is quite the reason for some of that weariness. On the off chance that we could truly feel enthusiasm what's more, truly feel as though we were really associated, maybe a great part of the anxiety that we have both been feeling of late would dissipate.

I think God needs you to live such a major life. God needs you to appreciate everything that He made you for, and I surmise that we're burglarizing one another of the endowment of enthusiasm that God put in us. Do you imagine that we could attempt to rediscover energy together? I know it's difficult, on the grounds that you sense that you don't have a sex drive. However, it's not just about sex; it's about feeling so near one another. That is the thing that I truly need. Would we be able to discuss how we can feel that closeness, that enthusiasm, that closeness? Also, how we can make it less demanding for you to feel it? Since that is the thing that I think our marriage needs.

As such, you're concentrating on closeness and cherish, and not on discharge. The discussion doesn't get to be about sex, or what you do in bed, or how regularly is sufficient. It concentrates on how we can feel love for one another and how we can truly encounter energy. Try not to contend about sexual discharge. Try not to contend about sexual needs. Try not to raise 1 Corinthians 7:5, about how your mate's body has a place with you. That won't likely offer assistance the circumstance (regardless of the possibility that it is valid). Rather, raise your longing for intimacy–a closeness that will engage you both, empower you both, and prepare you both to manage the world together. At the point when a couple is truly encountering that, they can tackle the world.

At that point the talk can swing more to overcoming barriers for sex, as I'm just as well tired, or I don't generally appreciate it, and you can begin taking a gander at how you can address these things to make closeness simpler. In the event that your life partner is anxious about it, you can discuss it lovingly, saying something like,

"I comprehend you're drained, yet I need a lot more for you. God made you carry on an enormous life, and I think He put me here to offer you some assistance with doing that. Would we be able to discuss how we can break through some of these issues?"

The fact of the matter is to make the subject of the discourse that you cherish your companion and you don't need them to pass up a major opportunity for intimacy—it isn't just about your sexual needs. It's about your needs as a couple.

Presently, a few individuals are certain to toll in and say that I'm by and large too simple on the life partner. In the event that they're not addressing needs, they're erring and they should be advised to get down to business. In a perfect world, we could simply say to somebody, "you're doing incorrectly", and they would stop. Be that as it may, I have once in a while witnessed that, in actuality. What I am proposing is to discuss it in a way that will probably get your life partner to comprehend your heart, and more probable to get your companion included in looking for an answer. What's more, to me, that is more imperative than telling your life partner that he or she isn't right and you are correct. In case you're not at the point where you can do that, and in case you're still excessively irate, then I'd recommend you chip away at your outrage before you carry any of this up with your partner.

Concentrate on Closeness in Different Ways

Closeness ought to be the fundamental center of your discussion with your life partner, on the grounds that as your mate perceives a more profound requirement for closeness, he or she will probably perceive to a greater degree a requirement for sex.

However, closeness is more profound than simply sex, and in the event that you deal with building closeness in different ranges of your life, you might just likewise fuel your companion's yearning for sex. So take a shot at your companionship. Get to know each other. Create leisure activities together. Take an enthusiasm for what your life partner is doing. On the off chance that your wife is overburdened with the house or with children, begin offering her all the more so she some assistance with canning unwind. In the event that your spouse is overburdened with work, do what you can to help him. Help one another quiet down, de-stretch, and invest energy together.

I have found that in my own particular life, as well. At the point when my spouse and I read Songs before we go to bed, or beg together before we go to bed, I'm generally more prepared to bounce him! So take a shot at creating profound teaches together. Go to chapel together. Perused the Book of scriptures together. In case you're uncomfortable begging so everyone can hear, get a book of supplications to God and read those (that truly is permitted). From multiple points of view, sex is a photo of our yearning for God; our aching to be profoundly associated and profoundly known. As we open ourselves up to profound enthusiasm, will probably feel different sorts of energy.

Seek after closeness in all aspects of your life: physical, social, and profound. And afterward converse with your life partner about how God needs you to lead lives of energy and closeness. That is His craving. On the off chance that we as a couple aren't encountering that, we're passing up a major opportunity for something excellent. So would we like to live little lives, or huge lives? Also, what would we be able to do to work towards that enormous life?

Chapter 3: The Male and Female Psyche

Men and women are built differently. Of course, you know that, but there is more to it than breasts and vaginas. A man is geared on testosterone, which is the male hormone. It is this hormone that is responsible for sex drive, for hair growth and the evolution of the masculinity of a man. He was the original hunter. He sees things in a very different way to his female counterpart. He is the provider. As long as he is providing, he feels happy enough. A woman, however, is geared by estrogen, which is the female hormone. She is likely to feel emotional and is the natural person to give care to children. You may not be that interested in the make-up of men and women and may simply have come here to see the positions that work, but you actually need to know these things because they come into play when you are making love.

Unless you have consensually agreed to basic sex without the emotions, a woman doesn't respond well to animal sex. There are certain things that a woman finds a turn-off, whereas men would not see them in the same way. One of these is the speed of sex. You need to appreciate that a woman needs to be coaxed into making love. That includes plenty of loving foreplay. This readies her for the sexual experience and helps her to become naturally lubricated for sex. Foreplay isn't just about lubrication. A woman sees it as being essential to sex because it shows a level of caring. She associates sex with love and affection, whereby a man may see it as a means to an end.

Thus, you need to remember that foreplay is part of sex and that this involves appreciating her. This may involve touching her breasts or kissing her neck, touching her clitoris and even indulging in oral sex. It makes her feel loved and when a woman feels loved, she is ready to give more than one who feels used. The foreplay also helps her to warm up to sex and you will find that women are equally giving on that front and that you may enjoy the foreplay yourself. Touching her skin and finding all of those sensitive areas may just be followed by her doing the same thing to you.

Experience of sex is gained through knowing your partner intimately. That means knowing all of the things that turn her on. Talk to her during lovemaking and make her feel like she has a voice. Often women don't say a lot in bed because the man tends to take over. If you allow her to participate, you will find that your own sexual experience and hers are likely to be much more satisfying.

I want you, in the spirit it was intended, to look at <u>a video</u> that is available on YouTube [https://www.youtube.com/watch?v=-qCouq-OIiM]. It will help you to see how relevant this book is about making your woman happy. In the video, men are asked to define where certain parts of the women's anatomy are. What they find is that none of them know. If you don't know where her G spot is, how can you satisfy it? If you don't know which part of the outer area of the vagina is her clitoris, how can you make her climax? The video is tongue in cheek but it demonstrates how men's ignorance of the female anatomy makes their sexual experiences a little hit and miss at best.

There are two areas on a woman, which produce orgasm. One is the G spot and one is the clitoris. The positions that you make love to making a difference to these being stimulated, as we will explain in our positions guide. However, during foreplay, these are areas that can really make her want hot sex. The G spot is located within the vagina and you may have to insert a couple of fingers to find it. If she is lying on her back when you insert the fingers, start to curl the ends of the fingers in the same way as you would if you were signaling someone to come here.

You will know the instant that you have found it from her labored breathing or her bodily response. The clitoris, on the other hand, is easier to find and lies at the top of the vagina if she is lying on her back. Move your fingers over the area outside her vagina until you feel a small lump. This area is the area where the clitoris is located. She may beg for more once you start, so be prepared to be very giving, indeed. It will help her lubrication, but it will also put her in the mood to experiment with sex and make your experience just as satisfying. Remember, the woman is the caring partner and once she sees the effort you are making to please her, she will be happy to please you in return.

Chapter 4: Sexless Marriage

Gravitation is not responsible for people falling in love. ~Albert Einstein

Sexual life can be durable in marital relationships. Experiences say, sexual gratification never ends especially in marital relations. You start your life with a sex night and continue it with having it daily. With an immersive marvelous, with sexual relation carry on even after having a couple of children or more.

And if we fall a look over another side of the situation then we will come to know about lack of intimacy in many marital relations. Here the point comes how is it possible that married couples lack intimacy? It can be well understood by the quote like:

"It is not a lack of love, but a lack of friendship that makes unhappy marriages."
— <u>Friedrich Nietzsche</u>

Yes, sexual relations is a product of many wondrous feelings, emotions, and sentiments. So, there can be a variety of reasons which can lead to a lack of intimacy in one's relation.

Reasons are on one side, now we will discuss about the solutions. What are the good solutions to boost up the level of intimacy between the couple? How to settle down the conflicts of sexless life in marital relations? Here are some good ideas:

Remove emotional distances:

A woman often remains reluctant to those partners who do to appreciate her. Such lack of appreciation gives her a feeling of lack of sexual intimacy.

Moreover, emotional stability doesn't only mean to have continued intercourse's, rather it means sharing of ideas, feelings, and tasks. Women feel more comfortable for the man who gives handy help to them even in the households.

So, if you are feeling sexual reluctance in your marital relationship then you must remove the emotional distances. Start sharing ideas with your partner. Help and support her in all of the emotional discords.

Do not step on the bed and kick start the sexual intercourse? Rather go on bed, talk with each other, share the daily routine, relax each other and then do whatever you want.

Admire each other:

Lack of intimacy means a lack of affection. And affection lacks where admiration lacks. Let say, the situation came where you do not even like the good thing of your partner because of marital discords. Then it's time to start admiring each other. You may start focusing on positives and avoiding the negatives of your partner. Show admiration in words and acts.

Let say, it's the day when your wife is making a hot Italian pizza for you, you may admire her by love words, by backing up with putting your hands in her hair and by eating the fast in company with her. Admiration is an immersive way of spitting the sexless life.

Make your figure appealing:

What you take by the term figure? It does not only mean to become hot and hot. Rather it means develop your physical appearance in accord with your partner's choice. If he loves slim and smarty ladies then follow a dietary plan and try to gain an ideal weight.

Try to make your appearance appropriate to the choice of your partner. And this rule is not only for girls.

Many of the time, men put on the weight, heavy their muscles and produce massive bearded and without caring what his mate wants. Get alarmed such all men and women. Just drop your breath and think for a while. I

If you do not like one thing in looks then how your mind will get ready to touch it and to indulge with it in physical relations. So, be careful in making the profile appropriate to one another choice.

Make sure to have safe environment:

Many of the time, trust breaks when a partner loses the level of security. Such a condition can come when the couple undergoes intercourse at a place like a hotel or at an unknown place. Any sort of crises like a police raid or a sudden attack form a stranger can develop the sense of insecurity even in the marital relation.

So, if you are feeling to have a lack of intimacy in your marital relationship then be the one to choose a safe environment. Never forget to lock the doors and the other openings of the room.

Moreover, keep secretes of your partner confidential. Let say, your partner is having some sort of sexual, physical, emotional or psychological issues, and then it is your duty to keep all of them really confidential. It will boost up the self-esteem of your partner.

Prioritize intimacy:

You can prioritize intimacy in many ways. Just like, when you and your partner approaches towards the bed, you may switch off the TV and stop their other extra activities.

Do not keep your partner on wait for hours and hours. Prioritize intimacy with your partner by spending about an hour or two before undergoing sexual intercourse.

Open the paths of communication:

Burst up the verbal as well as the non-verbal paths of communication. Try to understand the gestures of your partner. Just keep in mind, intimacy is something more important than the sexual intercourse.

Just going in bed and making wild tries is a foolish task. You can never get charm and joy from such a wildish strives. You may develop emotional understanding by enhancing the communication level between each other.

Extends the ways for joy able orgasm:

Sexual intimacy is something more chilly and frosty then that of other intimacy. Sticking to only one way and carry on doing sex, in the same way, will deduce the ejaculation and lubrication rather than enhancing them.

So, find various good ways of yelling the joy able orgasm. You can change the bed's positions, sex positions, and surrounding your bedroom. Moreover, you can also take help of the tactics like experimentation by doing role-playing, practices with orifices, doing some fantasies and taking the help of some sexual guides.

Add music:

Music is considered to be a soul of life. So, this life boosting serum can enhance the level of intimacy as well. If you are feeling you and your partner are having a low level of intimacy then make it sure to add music in your life. You can add pop music, fog music and so on in accord with your choice. You can also set down the music during the time of intercourse as well.

The above are all the golden ways of boosting intimacy in a sexless life. There is a huge link between intimacy and sexual life. If you think you will go under the blanket with anyone and you will feel love to undergo sex with him then you are damn wrong. Make reliable relations and then follow a guide to make your marital sex life better.

Chapter 5: Everybody's Different

Most of us have had reasonably varied sex lives, as modern people. Few of us come to marriage, or long term partnerships as virgins, unless we're either very young, or very cloistered. So it's clear that most modern adults know what it's like to have sexual experiences that are disappointing and unsatisfying. It's inevitable that this should happen when we approach sex as a sport, a diversion, or something to be pursued with little thought as to the spiritual nature of our sex partners. What could be more disappointing than sex that didn't make us feel connected to our partners?

But there are times when physical realities beyond anyone's control are what get in the way of satisfying sex. Sometimes, we end up in bed with people to whom we are not well-matched, physically. If we truly care about someone, we find our way around these physical realities. Interestingly, the Kama Sutra has a prescription for the physical statuses of men and women and about who fits best with whom. I'm sure you'll agree, after reading through the physical types laid out in Kama Sutra, that there is some logic involved. But our brief review must be read in the light of the sexual advice offered following this section, actually serves to mitigate the disparities described in terms of male/female genitalia.

Physical types

Kama Sutra sets out three categories of both men and women, concerning the various characteristics of their respective genitalia. I trust no one will personalize any of what's to follow. We're made the way we're made and (amazingly), one size does not fit all! In fact, there are physical types to which we're more suited than others, according to Kama Sutra. We all know how it feels to find a lover who "fits". We also know how to accommodate lovers who fit a little less perfect, through experience and the application of emotional tenderness and attachment.

Men are classified as hares, bulls or horses. I don't suppose anyone will have too much difficulty discerning what we're talking about here. We're talking about the size of what is called in the Kama Sutra the "lingam" (male genitalia). Of the three types, hares are the smallest and horses, the largest.

Women are classified as deer, hares, or elephants. These designations refer to the "yoni" (female genitalia) and refer specifically to depth. In Kama Sutra, the largest male size corresponds to the medium size in the female. In fact, the Kama Sutra posits that the male member determines the level of satisfaction in the female by being a little "too much". Many women will attest that size doesn't matter. This is, in fact, not only a bromide to soothe the frayed ego of males of smaller genital dimensions. It's true. The male member is only as good as its host's expertise. While the Kama Sutra doesn't mention this aspect of sexuality, I'd be more than willing to go out on a limb and guess that the information offered in the book concerning sexual congress is (at least to some extent) intended to mitigate the effect of "mismatched" genitalia.

Suffice to say that the physical typology of Kama Sutra, while an interesting artifact of the times it was written in, perhaps reflects a truth about the male authors that most women will readily recognize. Women know that the size of the lingam pales in importance next to the sexual expertise of their lovers. For this reason, it's important to read Kama Sutra in its setting and take from it that speaks most eloquently to us and our times.

Whether you're a hare, a deer, an elephant, or a horse, the appropriateness and harmony of your match has much more to do with your approach and interplay with your partner than it does with the size of your genitalia. I believe this assessment is more than fair and serves to perhaps soften the blow of the somewhat arbitrary genital typology offered in the Kama Sutra.

Levels of passion (libido)

We all have varying levels of need for sexual union. Even between loving partners, these levels can be at odds with one another. They're not static, though. Our libidos wax and wane, as part of the rhythms of our lives. There will be times when we're either both more inclined to our sexualities, less so inclined, or when we're at opposite ends of our respective libidinous arcs. The Kama Sutra also describes the various levels of passion and how they can be manifested in our sex lives.

Some people seem to have an endless amount of sexual energy. Others, very little. They tend to believe that sex isn't all that important. Others are between these two polarities. The Kama Sutra states that both men and women can fall into any of these three categories: intense, weak and middling. It further states that some go for the long game, others are satisfied in very little time and still others are of mediocre endurance. But the Kama Sutra all makes special provision for the very specific needs of women and actually puts them in the driver's seat in terms of sexual endurance.

Because women (for the most part) don't ejaculate in the same way men do, women take an entirely different approach to sexuality. This is, in fact, the model. During lovemaking, women feel pleasure as a more holistic experience, whereas men tend to focus on intercourse and the finality of their own orgasms. Because of this key sexual difference, women can reach climax, but continue to be connected to their partners physically and entirely invested in continuing the experience. Men, having reached ejaculation, tend to disconnect entirely – even fall asleep! This can be a bit of a problem for women who are interested in continuing the sexual encounter, once the man they're with ejaculates, rolls over the goes to sleep.

There is a biological reason for this male habit, one supposes, but it certainly doesn't serve the needs of the woman, which are paramount in the realm of making love.

The Kama Sutra's explanation for this variance between men and women is, once again, a product of the time in which it was written. There was little in the way of biological information available to people in those times. And so the Kama Sutra tends to cast the woman as emitting "semen" from beginning to end of any given lovemaking session. Of course, as modern people with access to information the ancients had no knowledge of, we know this isn't the case. All the same, it might have seemed a good explanation at the time, as men attempted to unravel the mysteries of the feminine.

It's for this reason that the Kama Sutra counsels sexual continence. This method sees the male withholding his own orgasm for the sake of prolonged lovemaking, in order that the highest quality of sexual union is reached. Women, the book notes, can be satisfied without a great investment of time, but this is not the desired type of sexual union. A truly transcendent sexual experience is prolonged, unhurried and exploratory in a highly sensual way. Sexual continence serves those seeking this type of sexual experience, as it calls on the man to be attentive to the quality of sex he's sharing with his partner and to put aside the need to climax.

But sexual continence doesn't *only* apply to men. It applies to women, also. Both partners seek to delay orgasm for as long as they can, in order to fully commune with one another physically, without feeling the pressure of orgasm. We all know that the orgasm is given an undue primacy in our sexuality. We feel it's the ultimate thrill. While there's nothing not to like about orgasms (let's face it), delaying them and learning to control them can lead us to an entirely different way of approaching one another sexually.

Delaying climax in both partners frees you to explore each other, without any presumptions about when the sexual encounter will end. Sexuality is not something that should be wedged in when there's time. Time is made for sexuality. Because of it's sacred, expressive nature, your sex life demands that you set aside time for it. If you find that difficult due to hectic schedules and family commitments, it's wise to start your journey toward a more satisfying sex life by sitting down together and choosing one day per week (to start) for physical intimacy. That means nothing can get in the way of what you've planned. You're free to spend as much time as you please, making love to one another, languidly and without any concern for when or how your session is going to come to a close. It will end when it's time for it to end.

Just setting the time aside can fill you both with anticipation and excitement. Agree with one another that the time you've set aside is sacred and that nothing will get in the way of it. Make it a special occasion. It gives a whole new meaning to the phrase "date night" and you'll probably find, once you've established the importance of this weekly special event, that you'll want to set another dayside. Perhaps two or even three. Practice makes perfect and the practice of sacred sexuality is no exception. If you intend to add sexual continence to your repertoire, you'll find that the more often you practice this method, the longer your lovemaking sessions will become. The sky is really the limit when you engage with each other on a level that transcends the procreative ejaculation, exchanging it for another type of orgasm entirely.

Chapter 6: How To Fall Back In Love With Your Partner

Do you worry that the spark has gone from your relationship and that, whilst you still love your other half, you are more like business partners or even roommates? This can be described as being emotionally divorced and in order to avoid this leading to actual divorce, the reasons behind this shift in feelings must be addressed.

By summing up your situation and coming to the conclusion that your life is infinitely better by having your partner in it, you are taking the first step to falling back in love with them. Of course, you will need to want to feel those feelings of love again and be positively inclined to revisit your former feelings.

Take a step back and examine the reasons you fell in love in the first place. Your partner had qualities that made you choose them as a mate, are those qualities still there? Have they changed or have they disappeared? By accepting that we all change over time we can sometimes expect too much from our significant others.

Physical, mental and spiritual changes are bound to happen and when we make our initial choice of partner we are unable to predict what form these changes will take. It is inevitable that life and its trials and tribulations will mold our personalities and bodies into a different person.

We also need to accept that not only have our partners changed but of course we have as well. Be honest with yourself and take on board your own shortcomings. It is very rare that the difficulties that arise are all down to one person, be honest about the strengths and weaknesses that you bring to the relationship.

The road to falling in love with your partner all over again starts with a full and frank conversation. Accept each other as you are, be strong enough to recognize each other's faults and weaknesses. Embrace your individual traits rather than viewing them as annoying habits!

Recognize that you are stronger together than apart. Are you better people because of your partner? Most loving couples are a strong unit and function better as a team. There is such comfort to be gained by knowing that if you are struggling with something you can turn to your other half and ask for help.

Stop focusing on what it is you find annoying about your partner and try and direct your energies to self-improvement. By diverting your attention and focusing on correcting your behavior towards your loved one you will see a change in your attitude towards them.

A loving relationship needs to be fought for. If one of you has already decided that the partnership is not worth the effort then you cannot change that. But if you are both committed to a future together then put on your battle gear and prepare yourself for some serious skirmishes!

Try to tell your partner what you value about your relationship. When you neglect the way you treat each other and stop caring about how you are acting you can create a vicious circle of resentment and hate. Be the first person to show the other undeserved loving feelings and create a way to break this cycle and regain that respect for each other and your feelings.

Is touching each other completely off the table? Bring back those special moments when your hands touch and you feel a thrill at having your partner close to you. Kiss for no reason, have long make-out sessions and feel like teenagers again! Do it in a way that leaves nothing to the imagination, you may feel a bit silly at first but you will soon forget that feeling when you are both left gasping for breath at the end of the kiss.

Planning for the future is a sure way of consolidating the fact that you can actually see a future for you both. Have you got into the habit of taking things for granted? Maybe you go to the same place for vacations every year and in doing so you have forgotten how exciting planning a vacation can be. Change things up a bit and plan a trip together, spend hours poring over brochures or searching the internet. Make sure the destination is one that you will both enjoy and will give you plenty of time to re-connect both physically and mentally.

By including your other half in all your future plans and dreams you are sharing the connection between your current life and your plans for your future. This is a great way to encourage the sharing of dreams and expectations and thus avoiding being too caught up in the realities of your everyday life.

If you do find it hard to implement these actions and maybe feel that the love is gone and past behavior cannot be forgotten and moved on from, this is troubling but not insurmountable. Marriage and relationship coaches are readily available. Counseling is also an option if you both refuse to let your relationship fail. Even when your partner is unwilling to work with you it is possible to seek counseling in order to change this mindset and create a desire to work out your differences.

Chapter 7: Talk Dirty To Me

Dirty talk can be good for any sexual relationship, from married couples to hookups. It's a great way to put some spice back into a relationship that has perhaps stagnated due to physical changes, children, work, busyness, or life in general. It's also perfect for turning up the heat with someone you've just started seeing. But dirty talk can be daunting, especially if you've never done it before. The things people say to each other (or think about each other) when they are turned on aren't things that are generally appropriate to say in public, so it's unlikely that you have a lot of practice saying them. And, just like any part of sex, what one person likes might not be what another person likes. When it comes to dirty talk, communication is key, both before, during, and after sex.

If you're brand new to dirty talk, a good way to start is simply to verbalize what you are already thinking or feeling. You've probably felt a strong desire for a partner, admired a physical characteristic of a partner, had an orgasm, or enjoyed a sexual act at some point--all without saying anything. Dip your toe into the world of talking dirty by telling your partner how you are feeling and what you are desiring. For the previous examples, you could try saying "I'm getting so turned on," "You have such an amazing butt, baby," "I'm getting close," and "I love what you're doing to me right now."

You can talk dirty in person, but you can also make good use of technology. For example, send a suggestive text to your partner as they are finishing up their day at work so they will be excited to come home to you and have some fun. Imagine their surprise when they pick up their phone and, rather than a message asking them to pick up some milk on their way home, they have a text from you saying, "I can't wait to taste you on my lips." If you're feeling really daring, you could even call them up for a little dirty conversation, perhaps asking what color panties they are wearing or telling them how much you're looking forward to taking off their necktie.

Don't hesitate to communicate with your partner about dirty talk. A conversation about what each of you prefers or is interested in before any dirty talk starts is a perfect way to avoid any awkward instances in the bedroom where one of you says something that is a definite turn-off for the other person. Some people prefer more clinical terms for their body parts, like "penis" or "vagina," while others find those terms to be too medical and would rather use "dick," "cock," "pussy," "cunt," or others. Find out what your partner likes and use their preferred term. The same rule applies for other dirty language. Some people are very uncomfortable with terms like "whore," "slut," or "daddy" during sex, while for others this type of dominant and submissive language is a huge turn-on. Others might prefer to come up with their own pet names to use during sex. Talk to your partner, and you won't find yourself saying "I want to fuck your pussy so hard" to a person who prefers "Honey, I want to make love to you"--or vice versa!

Dirty talk can also play an important part in fantasies and role-play sex. Most people have sexual fantasies, and it's common for people to develop fantasies that they routinely masturbate to. These fantasies might be scenarios that they would very much like to have happen in reality, or they may not actually be acts that the person would find particularly enjoyable. In either case, dirty talk can help people indulge their partner's fantasies during sex. For example, if one partner has a rape fantasy, the other could help indulge it by saying things that emphasized the first partner's lack of control, such as, "I'm going to take you, there's nothing you can do." It's highly unlikely that the first partner would want to be raped in reality, but in a trusting relationship, that fantasy can become a big turn-on through dirty talk. It can be difficult to tell your partner about your fantasies, and some people want to keep their in private. However, if it's something you want to share, it can create some great opportunities for steamy sex.

Role-play sex is similarly driven by dirty talk. Partners that are into role-playing may have costumes that fit their roles, but much of the atmosphere is created by the way they communicate. If a couple likes to play the roles of a school teacher and a naughty student, for example, they may dress accordingly, but much of the fun will come from the way the teacher talks to the student. "You've been a very bad boy and I'm going to have to punish you," and other phrases will drive him crazy. Talking dirty can also allow you to indulge in your role-play fantasies when you don't have costumes available, such as on vacation or when you don't want to spend money on elaborate setups. There's no limit to what you can create with words!

Communicating with your partner, figuring out what each of you likes, and starting to use dirty talk will raise the temperature of your relationship and keep you having more reasons to try out those sex positions in the first three chapters!

Chapter 8: How To Spice Things Up In The Bedroom

While knowing how to please your partner and how to please yourself is one of the most important aspects of a happy sex life, there are some tips and tricks you can use in order to spice things up a little in the bedroom. Follow some of these suggestions and you'll be pleasantly surprised!

Wear Red

Men are visual creatures and when they see a woman in red, they are turned on. The color red helps the men alter their perception of how attractive a woman is, but it doesn't change how they rate intelligence, personality, or competence. Men are more likely to want to have sex with a woman they were on a date with if she is wearing red. They're also willing to spend more.

Yoga

One study in India demonstrated that men who wanted to prolong their orgasms saw an improvement after they practiced yoga for an hour every day. The study showed that the men could actually triple the amount of time they lasted during sex after they took up yoga. It concluded that stretching and isometric holds during the exercises for the core strength and pelvic muscles helped them prolong their time until orgasm.

Be Vocal

Those who spoke up about what they want in the bedroom said they are more satisfied with their partner in bed. Those who talk about sex, when they are actually in the act, are more sexually satisfied. If you're afraid to talk about what you want, start with some non-verbal cues in order to signal to your partner what it is that will help you have a good time.

Comedy

Research has shown that those who visit comedy shows and laugh before they hit the sack are more likely to have higher blood pressure and their heart rate is increased. When the cardiovascular system is already working, your body is ready for pleasure.

Morning Sex

Men finish stronger and last longer in bed when it's in the morning. It's also really great for their overall mood and health, as well as for women, too.

Testosterone levels in men actually peak overnight, so men are the readiest to go in the morning. Between being rested and having high testosterone levels, they have more energy and can last longer between the sheets.

Exercise

Not only is working out great for men's physical appearance, but it's great for their stamina in bed. Men who exercise have been shown to experience fewer problems in bed. Those who are sedentary are actually at a higher risk of developing erectile dysfunction, and this can lead to some serious problems in the bedroom as well as out of it. Those who participate in cardio activity for twenty to thirty minutes daily are fifty percent less likely to experience erectile complications than inactive men.

Purple

Purple seems to be a color that boosts people's moods, whether they know it or not. Therefore, add a splash of purple to your room, maybe just a pillow, and you might notice an increase in your sex life!

Wine

Women who drink one or two glasses of wine on a daily basis actually have a better sex life than women who don't. A study in Tuscany demonstrated that women who drank had a more satisfying sex life compared to women who never drank. The study advised caution, though because women can experience sexual dysfunction in the bedroom with too much to drink.

Men Should Drink, Too

A study conducted in 2009 demonstrated that drinking enhanced men's performance during intercourse. This opposes the widespread belief that it hinders men in the bedroom. Those who drink on the weekend, are high-risk drinkers, and who exceed the alcohol intake guidelines actually experienced less erectile dysfunction. But the research cautions against binge drinking.

Try Something New

Doing the same old same old in the bedroom can get boring fast, so sometimes it's all about trying something new. People who have been together for a long time almost always fall into a rut at some point during their relationship, but it can be pretty tricky to get out of because women and men fear rocking the boat. But ladies, the change could be something as simple as different colored lingerie or a massage. Women and men could suggest using some toys or even just taking a shower together.

Chapter 9: Prepare Your Temple Of Love; Your Body

The path of tantric sex proclaims that your body is the temple of love. You have to ensure that you keep it healthy. You have to be fit in order to attain higher levels of ecstasy. This chapter gives you a few tips that you can use to keep your temple fit and healthy.

There are certain yoga positions that you can use to help facilitate the flow of energy in your body. The practices mentioned in this chapter are of great importance since they will help you channel and control your sexual energy.

We often take our body for granted. We do not worry about it and do not realize that it is the bridge to attaining bliss. You have to worship your body and treat it well in order to attain high levels of ecstasy.

Building love for your body through the looking glass

The most important part while preparing your body is to remove any negative thoughts that you have about your body. You have to view every part of your body and your private parts and see how good they are. If you feel that you are fat, you can tell yourself that you have curves. You must do this to ensure that you have fun during sex and that you are able to obtain pleasure.

Stand in front of a full – length mirror and remove your clothes. If you prefer it, you can do it after a bath. Look at every inch of your body. Start from your feet and continue to look upward. Reach the top of your head and stop. If you find yourself criticizing yourself, stop right there and give yourself a compliment. If you have said, 'My ass is fat', you can change that to, 'I have a full and luscious ass'. You should not worry about not telling yourself the truth. You are only shifting the focus and bringing a positive reaction.

Move on to observing your private parts – your genitals. You will have to focus on every aspect of them. You must look at the colors, identify how they are shaped and also observe the moistness in the areas. It is important that you do this in order to be more confident.

Observe your first chakra that is located at the base of your spine and the anal area. This is the chakra that provides you with a notion of security. You have to sit down and observe this area in the same way that you did with your genitals.

The connection between yoga and tantric sex

Yoga is one of the best methods to prepare your body. There are many tantric masters who have also mastered yoga. They have learned these poses for years together to ensure that they have control over their bodies. If you practice yoga, you will be able to control your mind and body. You will also be able to control the movements in your body. You will be able to achieve multiple orgasms and also control your ejaculations. This will benefit your overall experience and also your health. It also enhances the physical experience that you share with your partner.

Simple yoga movements

This section covers a description of the simplest yoga movements that you can perform alone! In the next chapter, you will learn about different exercises that you and your partner can perform together.

The head lift.

Ensure that you are standing straight! Tilt your head towards the sky. You should tilt it in such a way that a string from the sky was pulling it upward from your crown. Keep your mouth closed. You have to inhale through your nose alone. When you inhale, move your shoulder blades to the back like you are forcing them to touch each other. Exhale and hold your feet to the ground. It should feel like you have fixed yourself to the ground. Relax your stance and repeat the process.

The cobra – pose.
Lie down comfortably on the floor. Extend your body and ensure that your stomach is touching the floor. Place your hands under your shoulders. Close your arms with your elbows placed at the back. Lift your chest upward and move your head to form a curve. Ensure that you are looking upward. Relax your stance and repeat the process.

The cat – pose.
Once you have finished the cobra – pose. You should put your head down, and slowly rise up on your knee. Stretch your spine in the direction opposite from the direction in the cobra – pose.

The resting – pose.
Once you have finished your cat – pose, you will have to move back to the initial position of the cobra – pose. Stretch your arms outward. Breathe freely. Ensure that

your forehead is on the ground and your chest is touching your knees.

The food you eat is what defines you

Food is what provides your body with energy, which is its fuel. Hence it is essential that you pay close attention to the food you eat. You know that foods with a lot of fat are unhealthy for your body. You must never eat heavy meals since they affect your digestive system. You must ensure that you eat healthy in order to facilitate your journey on the path of tantric sex.

When you have a clogged drain at home, you will not have a free flow of water. In the same way, if your digestive system is clogged the flow of energy in your body is interrupted. You will have to cleanse your body of toxins occasionally. You can do this by eating raw fruits or going on juice fasts. But every approach is not right for you. What works for one will not work for another person. It is best to meet a nutritionist in order to identify the perfect diet for your body. You must ensure that this diet facilitates your journey.

Chapter 10: How To Reach Your Maximum Pleasure

In reality, the best way to reach your maximum pleasure is to know your body and help your partner know your body. You are ultimately the person who is responsible for your orgasm, not your partner. If you don't tell him or her how to help you get off, then they're not going to know if they're ever doing anything right. You don't want to fake and orgasm because that is the ultimate betrayal for some people. Imagine being with your partner for a year and finding out that all that time, they weren't enjoying sex with you as much as you had hoped they were.

So, this chapter is going to discuss the different positions that both women and men will enjoy during sex, and how each gender gets off.

Increasing the Odds of Orgasm in Women

Ladies, men want you to orgasm just as much as you want to orgasm. They are not having sex with you for their pleasure alone, but it can seem like that if you never tell them what they're doing wrong or right in bed. So the first thing to do is speak up and tell the man you're with that what he's doing is not doing it for you. Once you've done that, follow some of these suggestions to help both him and you bring yourself to orgasm.

There should be direct clitoral stimulation during intercourse. The woman or her partner should use one or two fingers and put a little pressure on the clitoral glans while having sex. Gently rub in a circular motion or back and forth. You can also use a small bullet vibrator on the woman's clitoris.

The best position for women is the woman on top position or cowgirl position because it allows the woman to easily access her clitoris and the man can reach up to stimulate her nipples. If the woman leans forward toward her partner's face, the pelvic bone of the man will stimulate her.

Some women prefer to stimulate their g-spot rather than their clitoris during intercourse. If you are that type of woman, you should let your partner know so that he knows how to please you. G-spot stimulation is different from clitoral stimulation.

There is currently a debate going on that the g-spot actually does not exist and that it's actually the inner roots of the clitoris being stimulated. Regardless of that debate, there are numerous positions that help women who climax by stimulating this area.

Positions that stimulate the side of the vagina that is closest to the belly button are best. Some manual stimulation or stimulation using some toys prior to intercourse is actually a good idea. The woman on top position is also great for g-spot stimulation because the shape of her partner's penis will stimulate the area.

Another position is reverse cowgirl. This is where the woman straddles the man with her back facing him. This is very useful if she's with a partner who has a penis that points downward rather than up.

In addition, putting a pillow under a woman's lower back while in the missionary position is another good way to get to the g-spot area. It angles the woman's vagina into a downward slant, making the area more accessible to penetration.

Having the woman lie face down with her body flat on the bed is another great way for the man to reach her g-spot. Experiment with depth and penetration with this position.

Positions that Satisfy Both Partners

You could find that if you're with more than one partner in your life, you're going to favor different positions with different partners. This is actually common and it's due to the fact that our bodies are going to fit together in a different way with different people. A position that you enjoyed with one person is going to be less enjoyable with another for many reasons. Deep penetration can be uncomfortable for some women, and yet men will enjoy positions that are deep because it allows for more thrusting. These positions are also likely to stimulate the entire shaft of the penis and offer an intense, varied stimulation for men.

If a man is looking for deeper penetration with his partner, he really needs to focus on the foreplay. There's actually a process that a woman's vagina goes through known as the tenting process. When she is aroused, really aroused, her cervix will actually extend back into the body and lengthen the canal. When the penis hits the cervix during intercourse, this causes pain for a woman. Ensuring that she is extremely aroused before penetration will ensure that she will not feel pain during intercourse.

Missionary position is actually the best position for this because women are able to control the depth of penetration by putting their legs flat or keeping them closer together. She can also widen her legs or raise her knees as her arousal increases and deeper penetration is acceptable.

The woman on top is also a really great position because it leaves the woman in control of how much penetration she receives. It also allows her to control the angle and the rhythm.

If you want to approach your partner about a sexual request, it's always best to be gentle. Be sure that you express how much you care for them and that you are happy with the sex life you have together but are curious about trying out something new. Sex should be a pleasurable, fun activity for everyone involved. So be sure to communicate honestly with your partner to let them know how a position feels for you. Variations of a position can always be made to make it pleasurable for both partners.

Chapter 11: Sex And Partner Bonding

This one's for all you partnered people. I know that not everyone reading is partnered, but if you're not now, you will be at some point, so read on.

Sex in a loving relationship is part of life. Many of us couple, whether serially or permanently and in those couplings, sex is a crucial ingredient in the couple's happiness.

The problem with sex and long-term relationships is that sooner or later, the bloom comes off the rose.

But that doesn't mean the wheels coming off the bus is going to be the next page you turn in your story.

The fact is, we become accustomed to each other. The thrill of newness fades (by most accounts, after the first 2 years) and we begin to neglect each other as sexual beings.

"But wasn't our attraction to one another what originally brought us together?" Some of us accept the "bed death" experienced in most long-term couplings without complaint, believing it's natural. Other have affairs. Still others look for answers. We ask ourselves if it's our fault. Do they not find us attractive anymore? Have we done something wrong?

Self-blame is an avoidance measure that allows us to blame ourselves rather than have a conversation with our significant other toward resolving the issue.

It doesn't have to be this way. Couples in loving relationships need to be vigilant about their sex lives together, honoring the reason they chose each other to begin with and continuing to express that love physically as the relationship continues.

A lasting afterglow

The Association for Psychological Science's journal, Psychological Science recently published a study implicating newlyweds.

The study revealed that following sex, partners enjoyed an "afterglow" which endures for 48 hours. This uplifting sensation is said to improve the quality of the relationship over time.

For two full days, partners feel elated and satisfied and that effect endures, strengthening the relationship by bonding partners together.

Here's something interesting – couples that reported a satisfying sex life in a long-term relationship didn't necessarily have sex every day. The long-lasting "afterglow" effect served to sustain the relationship sufficiently for couples having sex once or twice a week.

The study showed that the afterglow effect was responsible for fortifying the pair bond, keeping it robust by keeping sex alive in the relationship.

A metaphor for intimacy

Intimacy isn't solely expressed in our sexuality. In fact, sometimes sex feels like one of the least intimate things in the world, as commodified as it's become in our society.

But in the context of a bonded pair, sex serves as a metaphor for intimacy. Most of us think of sex as the ultimate physical expression of love. In fact, when it's approached as an act, which reinforces the connection between two people, it becomes exactly that.

By connecting with each other physically, bonded couples commune with each other on the physical, intellectual and spiritual level. As their bodies move in physical desire, so their spirits speak to one another and their intellects share secrets, renewing the basis for the relationship.

Affection and sex go together. Even fleeting sexual encounters have an element of affection. The touch of a lover and being naked and free with another person has a profound effect on the resiliency and quality of the relationship.

Have more sex

People tend to get clammy when it comes to bringing up sex in their relationships. They don't want to hurt their partner and they don't necessarily want to rock the boat (in a bad way).

But revising sex in your relationship renews, refreshes and strengthens it, so it's well worth your time. Here are some great ways to have more sex.

- If you're thinking your partner "isn't into it," ask yourself why? Is that coming from you? Have you made your approach? Make it and make it sexy.
- Make dates for sexual intimacy. Take your time and make an event of it, bringing out your favorite tricks and sexy surprises.
- If either of you is experiencing sexual dysfunction, talk about it. Then talk about ways around it. All

sex isn't penetrative. There are so many ways you can get around issues of dysfunction and still have great, pair-bonding sex.

- Stop overthinking it. To have great sex, it's important to turn off your preoccupations, resentments and other potent players in your head. Let your body do your thinking for you. It's sex, not chess!
- And remember – orgasms are the final act. If all you're going to think about is getting to the punch line, then it is doubtful either of you will enjoy getting there.

It's about the journey, not the destination, so put the orgasm in its proper place and make your sexual encounters last. Make them fun and detach that final act from the beautiful story your bodies are telling together.

- Touch each other more often. Spend time looking into each other's eyes, especially while you're talking. Be attentive to one another and spend time appreciating your partner.
- Dress up for each other. Like setting aside time for sexual intimacy, it's also important to present yourself to your partner in a way that honors your reverence for each. Talk to your partner about date

nights that don't necessarily involve sex, but demand that you dress beautifully for each other. Then take each other out to dinner, a show, or another event and share your mutual admiration with the world. Conspiring to show one another off is not only fun, it's sexy!

- Build anticipation into your schedule. Planning your "play dates" should also draw on the bliss of impatiently awaiting the night (or day). Send him a new pair of his favorite style of underwear in a wild print or color, with a note saying you'll see them on the appointed date. Send her a new sex toy (or flowers, depending on who you are and what your personal seduction style is). Have fun working each other up into a lather!

Being together isn't just about sharing the rent or having children. Romantic partnerships are formed to honor a love, which has created a new entity in the world. That's you two.

That new entity needs to be nurtured, fed and watered and sex is a tremendous nutrient required for it to truly thrive (and survive).

So, take your sex positive attitude and live it out in your relationship. Be open with your partner. Be fun.

Be affectionate. Be united in your demand for a stronger bond between you.

Add more sex and develop that life-long love that's evergreen.

Sex may not be the same thing as love, but it's one of romantic love's great joys. Let it out to play more often. Be happy. Be loving. Be sex positive.

Chapter 12: Stages Of Sexual Arousal In Humans

The following are some moves you can do on your women to get her engine purring! These techniques are actually from woman who secretly told what they like! Experiment with your woman and see what hit's her hot spot!

The Sensual Touch

Before having sex, stand in front of your woman after she undresses. (help her undress as it builds anticipation) Hold your fingertips just above her skin. Lightly brush her hair back. The large part of your fingers should be hovering above her skin. You can switch it up now and then with your nails slightly touching here. Move your hand slowly and sensually up and down her body. The sensation will drive her wild. Anticipation is a big turn on for women. By lightly brushing your fingers above her skin so that they gently touch her body hairs, you can send shivers up her spine and caress her body.

The Teasing Lick

Instead of going straight for the sucking on the nipples, take your time and build the tension. Make a circle round her breast with your tongue or finger before going for the nipples. This works because of the sensitivity radiates out from a woman's hot spots. The surrounding tissue around the nipples is very sensitive to a woman. Start where her breast starts to rise from the chest. Slowly circle your way up with your finger or tongue to the nipple. Once you make contact with her nipple, sensually bite or suck it good. To tease her more, just as you brush up against her nipple spiraling up, pull out again for another sensual licking spin.

The Lick Blow

Lightly lick her neck, genital area, nipples, or sensitive areas on her body. You can get these areas wet with water or alcohol. Simply swish some of your mouth and lick the area you like. Then lightly blow on the wet patch followed by a slow sensual lick. Repeat to drive her crazy. This can send shivers down her spine! It works because of the contrast you are creating between hot and cold, hard and soft. The further apart the sensation is in contrast, the more intensity she will feel.

The Oral Flick

When she's almost climaxing through oral sex, quickly give her flick on the clitoris with your tongue. It would be best if you made sure the clitoral hood is out of the way for better pleasure. Be gentle and pull the hood out of the way if you need to, and make quick motions with your tongue up and down the clit. Most men make the mistake thinking the clit is just tiny nerve ending in a small area in her body. By doing the oral flick you cover more area and create vibrations that carry the sensation beyond your tongue's reach.

The One-Two Combo

While nibbling and sucking on her erect nipples, you play with her clitoris with your fingers. The sensory combination will get her juiced up. Don't be surprised if she starts to puts her leg over your side; she may be signaling for you to go deeper. There's a direct sensory connection between her clit and nipples. Lightly biting and teasing her nipples can create tingling in her clit.

The Suck and Seal

While licking her nipples, change it up and suction your lips around her nipples. Create a good seal with your lips and inhale and exhale to create a vacuum and put pressure on her breast. Take the air in through your nose and breathe through the mouth, then suck in with the mouth. It can create a pleasurable feeling for her. You are using the sensation of contrast for her. Like hot and cold, you are now using the push and pull effect, which can double her pleasure.

The Oral Finger Combo

While licking her clitoris and you get her stimulated, insert your finger in her vagina and give her some good firm strokes. As she is about to orgasm, try inserting more fingers to give her more to pulse against. This combination can feel great for her. The vagina and clit are on different nerve networks, so they can trigger separate sensations. By doing a separate combo on the vagina and clit, you can double her pleasure! Some women like the pleasure of being filled up during an orgasm, so inserting more fingers while she climaxes can give her the sensation she wants.

The Slow Thrust

Kiss her neck or lips, pause a couple of seconds and enter her slowly bit by bit. Resume your thrusting in gradually for intensity. This works because you are adding variety to your thrusts and it keeps her guessing. Stopping and starting builds on a former sensation, and it lets you jump and skip to the different pleasure levels.

The Missionary Dive

While having sex in the missionary position, push yourself forward on the balls of your feet and toes so you are humping her high. Your hipbone should be close above hers. Then thrust into her at a downward angle very slowly. You can give her explosive orgasms this way. This is works because during sex her clit will typically gets neglected. By changing up the angle, your penis shaft can get direct contact with her clit and give it the stimulation it needs.

The Pillow Boost

When you're about to penetrate her in the missionary position; put a pillow behind her back where her lower back and butt meet. Let her adjust until she's comfortable. This will tilt her in a way that your thrusting will give her a different sensation. Don't be surprised if your thrusting gives her deep pleasure and she reaches orgasm faster. Angle makes a big difference in your penis thrusting into her. At the right angle, you could be making contact with her G-spot.

The changed angle of her pelvis makes contact with sensitive spots like her clit more reliable.

The G-spot Push

As you having sex and thrusting away, put your hand below her belly button. This can give her an intense orgasm because it helps expose the G-spot. When she screams with ecstasy, you know you're in the right spot. Many women don't mind this because it only lights up during firm pressure; which most women don't get during sex.

The Head Rush

Position your woman so that her head and shoulders are dangling over the bed. You can turn her sideways on the bed if you have to. Then thrust into her as her head dangles and blood pours in, and oxygen is depleted. For some women, the intensity of the head rush with the physical thrusting can increase the pleasure of orgasm. Stop if you see her get too light headed. The last thing you want is your woman to pass out during sex! Penetrate her slowly as she dangles and see her squirm with pleasure.

The Rocking Chair Thrust

Use a rocking chair or recliner as you penetrate her. Have her lie on her back, and you kneel below her and thrust. Use the rocking motion of the chair to get her going with more pleasure. The rocking motion adds to the flavor of your thrusts. Since you are at a slightly lower angle than her from the chair, you can be hitting her G-spot with your penis as you rock along. You might surprise her with your creativity using this move.

Chapter 13: Ways To Make You Last Longer In Bed

So, this is more of a recap with a few new ideas thrown in for good measure. At the end of the day, most men want to be able to last longer in bed, not just those who suffer from premature ejaculation. We all know it isn't any fun for either of you when things end too quickly but, on the other hand, all the media hype that says you should be going at it for half an hour or more is also wrong. Many men are conscious of the fact that they may be finishing just a little too quickly for their partner as all those Hollywood movies and magazines would have you believe women love sessions that go on for hours.

That is all complete and utter rubbish and nothing but hype. That said, there are times when you could do with lasting just a little longer than a few minutes so here are some killer tips to help you hold back for longer:

1. Back to your teenage years

Remember how, as a teenager, you used to spend what felt like hours kissing and making out without actually having sex? Felt good, didn't it. So, go back to doing that. Spend more time on kissing your partner, on exploring each other using your hands and your mouth before you even think about actually having sex.

2. Learn how to massage

When you lead a busy life, it becomes quite difficult to find the time for sex and it isn't easy to make the move from your busy working life to a sexy erotic one. Stress is the culprit here and before you can even begin to feel like getting down to it, you need to de-stress. The very best way to do that is through massage, and if you do it properly, both you and your partner will be completely turned on by it. You do need to learn how to do this properly, though; if you don't you can actually cause more problems. Learn to give a very deep and satisfying massage and then each of you takes about 5 or 10 minutes to massage each other before you think about sex. Not only are you really getting in the mood but you will be helping each other to breathe properly and to relax. Foot and back messages are perfect for priming you for pleasure and comfort and, think of it this way – each minute you spend intimately massaging your partner is another minute towards your goal of lasting longer in bed.

3. Take it in turns

Most sexual sessions are pretty much a give and take pleasure method, in which each of you touches each other at the same time, which means you are both heading for the finish line pretty darn quick. There is a golden rule here if you really want things to take longer – take it in turns to touch each other. From now on, let your partner do the touching while you relax, lie back and take as much pleasure from it as you can without getting too over-excited. Then return the favor; let her lie back while you do the touching and exploring. Both of you need to learn how to use your hands properly to give as much pleasure as possible, leading both of you down the road to arousal but not so quick as it would normally happen.

4. Control your surroundings

The truth of the matter is when you are in a comfortable position, in comfortable surroundings, a place where either you or your partner is likely to get too over excited, you are more likely to last longer in bed. Don't be tempted with public sex or anything else that could be just that little too exciting for you. If your most comfortable place for sex is in bed then keep it in the bedroom, at least until you have learned how to control your orgasm.

5. Woman on top

I mentioned this one earlier; by having the woman on top, you don't feel so stimulated. Plus, ask her to take it slowly. Long, hard and fast thrusts are pretty dangerous for a man on the edge! You could also try penetrating her and then not moving for a couple of minutes, just to let yourself get acclimatized to her.

6. Use the start-stop technique

With this technique, your woman will stimulate you until you start to get close to an orgasm. At this point, tell her that she must stop. When your levels of sexual tension have reduced, it could be as quick as 15 seconds, start again. By doing this frequently, not only will you last longer for that particular session but you will also begin to understand your own feelings and will learn how to stop yourself.

7. Learn to breathe from the belly

When you breathe deeply, it is actually a direct correlation to ejaculation. So, breathing deeply and slowly should help you to reduce stress and anxiety, thus slowing down your rate of ejaculation. Learn how to breathe so that your belly will rise before your chest does and practice this in conjunction with the start-stop technique. You could also practice the yoga breathing technique I told you about earlier.

8. Read the Kama Sutra

Preferably together as this will heighten the pleasure for both of you. Plus, you could always try out some of the positions! In all seriousness, though, there is a specific technique that is mentioned that can help you to stay the distance. Using this technique, start off very slowly, with just one in and out stroke per three seconds. Then you can begin to build up the strokes, adding in more, over a session of about four or five minutes until you are at the stage where you are giving one stroke per second. If you feel as if you are about to lose control, stop, stay inside your woman until you regain control and then start from the beginning again

9. Out of your head

And I do not mean on drugs or alcohol! One of the biggest killers during sex, the one thing that will affect whether you can maintain an erection or not, is stress. And that comes down to what is going through your mind. In the case of premature ejaculation or in those who seem to rush it all the time, the main thoughts are going to be on your abilities and your performance and that will likely push you over the edge. Learn how to change your thinking to positivity and confidence pushing worry and stress out of the way. If you start to feel anxious or stressed during sex, stop, breathe deeply and then focus on your inner self. Get rid of the negative thoughts and put your attention firmly on you and your feelings.

10. Try new positions

I gave you five positions to try earlier to help you last longer in bed but you could always open that copy of the Kama Sutra. There are specific positions that are designed to make your orgasm happen quicker and others, like the ones I told you about that will prolong things. Experiment, try a few out and see what works and what doesn't.

11. Learn to control your ejaculatory muscle

When you ejaculate, do you ever wonder what physically causes it to happen? There is a specific muscle that controls your ejaculation and, when it is relaxed, you simply cannot ejaculate, no matter how hard you try. We talked about it earlier – it's called the PC muscle and it what is responsible for letting the semen come out when you come. To control your rate of ejaculation, you have to know how to control this muscle. Practice the exercises we talked about earlier as much as you can until you have almost full control over it. This won't be instant; it can take as much as four weeks to get really good results. It will also take a great deal of regular practice to get it right and become a sexual master.

12. Learn to control your confidence and mental health

Back in the olden days, it used to be thought that premature ejaculation was the result of mental health problems and men who suffered from it were immediately sent for hypnotherapy or to see a psychiatrist. Obviously neither of those worked very well. While premature ejaculation is a physical condition, it is also linked to mental health and this must not be ignored. You must learn how to manage your concentration levels, your thoughts, and your confidence levels while you are having sex. If you don't, it will have a serious effect on how long you can manage to last for.

13. Masturbate often

If you truly want to know how to last a long as possible between the sheets, you need to get more in tune with your own sexual responses. To do that, you're going to have to masturbate more. When you begin to stimulate yourself, make sure that you stop before you can't. Let's say that, on a scale of 1 to 10, the orgasm is number 10. So stop yourself at about 8. Make sure you leave time to calm down and then start again, working your way back up that scale. Do this as often as you need to in order to learn how to control yourself.

14. Learn how to cool down

Whether you suffer from premature ejaculation or not, you should still learn a few methods for cooling down. You can practice these so that, if you do find yourself heading towards being out of control you can stop yourself before you do go over the edge. Do your research and find the methods that will work for you, that will help you to last a bit longer in bed.

15. Change it up

What is the absolute best thing you can do when you find yourself heading fast toward that point of no return? The biggest piece of advice that I can give you is to change your speed. Men should have a go at teasing their partners; remove your tool from inside her and rub the head up and down over her sex. There are a lot of nerve endings there and this will make her feel great, as well as help to slow you down a bit.

16.   Squeeze

Earlier on, we mentioned the most sensitive parts of the penis. There are three areas that, when squeezed, can help to slow you down and keep you hard. First, when your penis is erect, make a ring with your index finger and your thumb around the base of it and squeeze it. This stimulates a ring around the base of the penis which helps to keep the blood where it should be. The second place is underneath the head of the penis. Applying pressure there can work wonders as it is the hot spot in most men and is full of nerve endings. Lastly, the perineum, the spot that is located in between the anus and the base of your testicles.

All of these techniques are designed for you, with you in mind. Obviously, you don't need to do all of what you have learned in this book, just what you feel comfortable doing, what makes you and your partner feel good and what works. Basically, do whatever it takes to make your bedtime sessions last as long as you both want them to.

There is something here that I must reiterate. You may think that it is OK to go for hours in bed and that maybe what you are aiming for. Please don't. Unless your partner is a machine or made of some other substance than blood, skin, and bone, it isn't wise or pleasurable to make sex last for a prolonged period of time, especially not the penetration part of it. It can be painful and uncomfortable, not just for your woman but for you too. Too much thrusting away can cause lubrication to dry up and then it becomes less of the pleasure and much more of the pain. You aren't in the movies and you don't need to perform for the cameras, just for you and her.

Chapter 14: Premature Ejaculation

Premature ejaculation is an issue for a lot of men and affects both male and female partners in different ways, leading to an inactive or unhappy sex life. The problem with premature ejaculation is in its very definition itself – how do you know your ejaculation is premature? What is the right time to have an orgasm exactly? There aren't any clear answers, but medically speaking, we define premature ejaculation as an orgasm that happens with minimal stimulation to the penis. Obviously, that could mean that the longer you abstain from sex, the faster you end up coming simply because even a little stimulation is too much stimulation. So you see where the issue starts – most men, at some point in their life, have experienced it. However, when it persists chronically, that's when it becomes an issue. We have already seen how, by practicing tantric sex and working with your chakras, you can harness your sexual energy and try to prolong your sexual intercourse and make it fun. But there are other, proved ways to help with the problem of premature ejaculation, both medical and non-medical.

Self-Treatment (Differentiating between Orgasm and Ejaculation)

The biggest problem men face when it comes to sex is that they can't differentiate between orgasm and ejaculation. The common perception of orgasm in society is that you hurry towards an ejaculation that bombards out of you; in reality, the ejaculate is the final orgasm for the male who can multiple dry orgasms before he finally lets the semen out. Orgasms and ejaculations happen one after another in rapid succession – the former starts before the latter and tapers off somewhere in the middle of ejaculation, which is why most people confuse the two terms. This means that like women, men can also be multi-orgasmic. In Tantra, we believe that a man directs his Kundalini through every chakra, slowly allowing the sexual energy to climb up, thus letting him experience a full-body, dry orgasm before he ejaculates. In any case, to help control premature ejaculation, you need to be able to differentiate between the two. Here's how - there is the pubococcygeus muscle or the PC muscle, which stretches from the pubic bone to the tailbone. Controlling this will help you control your ejaculations to a point. To identify if this muscle is strong or weak, you must try to stop your urine-flow mid-stream while peeing; it sounds icky, I know, but this is good for your sex life! A strong muscle will help you stop your pee stream, and is good for control of your ejaculation – if it's weak; you need to be able to control it.

So to help with your premature ejaculation, here's what you do –

Get inside the bathroom and start masturbating.

When you feel like your climax is close, stop. Contract your PC muscle and hold it tight to a count of 10.

Let go and breathe slowly; take a minute to regroup and start masturbating again – you'll find that your climax isn't coming as fast as you'd expect it to!

As you get closer to your climax, you'll notice that at the base of your penis, you're experiencing smaller contractions. This is when you're about to ejaculate – squeeze your PC muscle when these tingles start in your pelvic cavity and stop stimulation. A few drops of ejaculate may slip out anyway, but you'll notice that the orgasm isn't as powerful as a normal climax is and that you're still hard. If you weren't able to stop ejaculation, it could because your PC muscle isn't that strong yet or that your timing of squeezing it was off. In either case, all you need to do is keep practicing – in fact, get your partner to join you in mutual masturbatory sessions to heighten the experience! It'll bring you closer because you're willing to trust them with an issue that's so personal and it'll boost your sex life because mutual masturbation is a kink most people have!

Psychological Help and Sex Therapy: A major reason for premature ejaculation is stress or depression and anxiety. You may have some problems in the beginning, as an inexperienced person, or someone who's abstained for a long time or you're just finding your footing – however, as you keep losing out, again and again, you end up getting performance anxiety and worry about satisfying your partner and in turn, your problem becomes worse. Since the exact cause of premature ejaculation is still mysterious, given that we can't even define premature ejaculation all that well, a solution is hard to find. What we do know is that the more anxious you get about not ejaculating prematurely, the faster your climax hits – it becomes a self-fulfilling prophecy 80% of the time. Overall stress or anxiety, not just about this, but life in general, can also lead to it. Going in for counseling to help you get back on the proverbial horse is an excellent idea. Premature ejaculation could be indicative of a bigger problem; perhaps you're depressed, or your marriage isn't satisfying or anything else. Going to a therapist to help you find out where you're losing out on life and then sorting that out could go a long way in helping you boost your sex drive. Another medical intervention would be to approach a sex therapist. Now sex therapy has more or less the same squeeze-control exercises that I've already mentioned, so you could try those first and then get more help from a certified sex therapist. They will put you -through a series of things such as mind and body control exercises, breathing exercises, focus exercises and the like – all are geared towards helping you understand and controlling your body better, which in Tantra, we already do.

Drugs: There are certain drugs that help with premature ejaculation, but you must be cautious when you take them since they could have several side effects. There are drugs known as serotonin reuptake inhibitors, the SSRIs like dapoxetine, which helps in ejaculatory delay. But they cause other sexual dysfunction such as erectile dysfunction, low libido and the like, so consult your doctor before you take any of these. Medicine for premature ejaculation is available, but medications that will help you get over premature ejaculation long term, without side effects, is still quite rare. The best way is to get to simply strengthen your core muscles and understand why you're experiencing it; getting stressed out because you're having a few early climaxes could be the reason why you're getting those orgasms in the first place! Be patient, be open to new ideas and communicate with your partner – this is the best way of overcoming premature ejaculation!

Chapter 15: How To Re-Light The Spark – 15 Ways To Fall Back In Love

Here we will go through **15** ways to relight that spark that you and your partner once had. Remember that feeling when you first got together? Yeah? That's what we're talking about. By following these steps, you will be able to enjoy a better sex life with your partner and fall back in love all over again.

Take some time to talk with your partner.

Sex is about communication. If you want to make a positive change in your sex life you need to feel comfortable talking to your partner about it, and you'll both be grateful for it. Tonight, take 15 minutes to sit down with your partner to discuss the plan and make it work for you! Everybody's different and sometimes a compromise might be the best way forward to jumpstart what each of you want to get out of the experience. Maybe you could go for a brief walk or have a quiet chat before turning off the lights, whatever feels more comfortable.

Continue to make time to talk each night. Having a daily check-in with your partner is, without doubt, the best way to make sure you're both happy with where things are going and that you're comfortable – make time for each other's needs. As well as helping keep things going, you'll feel more and more connected on a personal level each and every time you have the chat which will naturally bring you closer together.

Make your own goals.

Ultimately, by the end of the next 2 weeks, you want your sex life to be better, but that doesn't mean that you can't take much more away! Improving your sex life involves your mind, your body and the relationship. You want to become closer to your partner, you want to feel sexier, you want to know that's how your partner feels too. Find the courage to ask your partner how they feel about the plan; what do they want to get out of it? Make a sexy goal to achieve – take your sex life to the next level. Approach sex with a positive attitude and mindset and see the results for yourself.

Ask yourself, what do I love about my body?

A lot of confidence in the bedroom comes down to self-esteem – how you genuinely feel about yourself: body and mind. What makes you feel beautiful? The truth is, body embarrassment should have no place in the bedroom and your sex life. When it comes down to it, you should love yourself and your partner will love you no matter how you feel about your body. Learn to love who you are and what you look like. Write down 5 things about yourself that you like, 5 reasons why your partner is attracted to you. Work on having a positive view of yourself. Build your self-esteem because there is no reason why you shouldn't feel confident in bed.

Have a long morning with your partner.

Stay in bed this morning. Turn off your 8.30 am alarm and take some time to just stare into each other's eyes, smile, cuddle. Talking isn't the only way to communicate with your partner, so make the most of every moment you have to show each other how you feel.

Say goodbye. Properly.

For most people, a simple 'goodbye' or a peck on the cheek has become normal before heading off to work in the morning or going out for the evening – it has become routine like brushing your teeth or brewing a morning coffee, but it really shouldn't be. Goodbye is a time to show your partner how you feel and make them remember you for the rest of the day. Take time to say goodbye before you or your partner leave for the day. Have a long, passionate kiss. Implement passion throughout your day and get the passion back.

Make the bedroom a place for sleep and sex.

Your bedroom should be made for nothing else, but for sleep and sex. Get away from other distractions like TVs, phones, and technology. Make your bedroom place that you look forward to going to. All it might take is some nice and new bedsheets and some new pillows. Make sure you make the bed every morning and get rid of clutter or mess. Keep your room tidy.

Have some alone time.

Ironically, rekindling a sexual connection with your partner might mean spending some time by yourself! Self-esteem is an important element to confidence in the bedroom and is an essential element to having great sex. You need to be comfortable with yourself, so spend time with yourself. Walk around the house naked, look at your body in the mirror when you're getting dressed, explore your body and rediscover what feels good. Caress yourself in the shower and in bed – learn more about yourself. There's nothing to ashamed of.

Exercise.

Healthy people have better sex. Period. Those who are physically active enjoy sex more and want to have sex more. Your self-esteem will skyrocket once you start an exercise regime, even if it is just 30 minutes a day. Your partner will be grateful for it too!

Try yoga.

Yoga has become more and more popular in the mainstream market, and for good reason. Yoga can help increase your self-awareness, flexibility and circulation – all things that are good for a healthy sex life. Even if you're new to it, start slow and learn the basics. It might even turn in to a hobby. You could even try and see if your partner wants to join in and try it with you.

Date night.

Date nights are brilliant. They help people reconnect, they relieve stress that built up over the week and increase attraction. A date doesn't need to be extremely expensive or extraordinary either, you just need to spend some quality time together. Put some thought into the planning too. Maybe you spend the night going to the restaurant you went to on your first date? Or maybe you want to try something completely new? This can help make new bonds with your partner – new experiences release chemicals like dopamine and make you feel just like you did when you first started dating.

You might want to take turns planning date nights for each other – show each other how much you care. Talk about this one with your partner.

Hit the gym.

Taking a session at the gym can really boost your endorphins. It can also help with male arousal problems which are quite common. Inactive men are up to 60% more likely to experience erectile dysfunction so try and get your partner to come along with you and invest in an exercise routine. Research has also shown that couples feel more attracted to each other after exercising and sexual arousal increases. It also helps to relieve stress – a common reason why people don't feel like having sex or showing physical affection for their partners.

Take a rest day.

Most people spend their days off doing chores or running errands for other people, but you need a day off! Turn off your phone and spend the whole day to yourself or with your partner. Lounge around and relax. Do nothing else.

Take a day away.

Taking a vacation can relieve all the stress in your life. Sometimes you just need an escape. And the best thing is it doesn't need to be anywhere exotic. Even taking a night away at a hotel can help couples feel like they're on a real vacation. And what's more? 'Vacation sex' is the ideal way to get that spark back to the relationship.

Have a laugh together.

After your chat tonight put on a funny movie or play a game that you both enjoy. Laughter is one of the best ways to connect with, and stay connected with, your partner. Laughter shows a genuine connection that can't be forced or made up – laughter is real in a relationship. Laughter is about connection. Sit together, make out, hold hands. Be together.

Show your partner some appreciation.

A compliment can go a long way in a relationship. Even the tiniest comments can make someone smile and relieve the stress that's built up. You might want to remind them that you're grateful that they are going through the plan with you. Remember, it might not be the easiest thing for them to be comfortable with! Show them affection and they will show it back.

Treat yourself.

Sticking to a plan like this can be quite demanding to begin with, so reward yourself! Buy yourself something sexy for tomorrow's date. Get some new lingerie or some makeup, whatever makes you feel better about yourself.

Date night.

Time for another date. Remember, if you planned the date last time, let your partner plan it this time. It's not a competition, but try and be thoughtful towards one another. Keep them going at least once a week and keep them fresh and exciting – they shouldn't be a chore! You should both look forward to spending the evening with each other. You could even save up to go somewhere a bit nicer once in a while.

Have a massage.

Physical contact stimulates the release of oxytocin – the more that's released, the more desire a woman will have. It may cost a little to get done, but once in a while you will reap the rewards.

Back to foreplay.

Don't forget about taking a night off from sex and focus on foreplay. For a lot of people foreplay is more pleasurable than sex altogether and feel closer after having it. And it's not all about receiving! 70% of men say that they enjoy giving oral sex to their partners, not just receiving it! So, make an effort to do it. The goal doesn't always need to be intercourse.

Another day, another rest.

Time to take one final rest day to reflect on everything that has happened. Do whatever you feel like doing whether on the list or not, with or without your partner. Today is about you and you need to make the most of it.

Chapter 16: Sexual Role-Playing Games

Sex doesn't always have to be serious. Sex can be fun, too. In fact, laughter and a sense of play helps break the tension during new sexual experiences. Playing games and goofing around will bring you both out of your shell, allowing you to try new things and push each others' erotic boundaries comfortably.

Silent Sex

Sounds easy, right? Wrong. Try making love to your partner without making a sound. Do what you have to do: bite your lip, cover his mouth, shove her face into a pillow...all is fair game. To ramp up the stakes, whenever one of you makes a noise – the other person has to totally stop what they're doing.

You'll discover that when you're not allowed to express yourself verbally or vocally, you find another way to let that pleasure out through biting, squeezing, and desperately grabbing your partner to fuck you deeper.

Sex Dice

Your sexual experience is all up to fate with a roll of the dice.

Each set comes with two dice. One lists different activities like "lick", "tickle", "squeeze" and the other lists body parts like "nipples", "ass", "belly button". This is a fun game to play with a glass of wine on the living room floor and watch where it leads.

Edging

When a vampire wants to turn human into a vampire, he must bite them without killing them. He must show extreme self-control and stop just before the human dies. You can think of Edging like this...without the whole death thing.

Edging is the act of coming so close to orgasm and then stopping. You repeat this over and over (3-4 times minimum) during the course of a few hours. When you finally let yourself or your partner cum...the orgasm will be one of the most intense you've ever had.

Make Bets with Dirty Wagers

Inject your sex life into everyday activities. When you're out and about, make sexy wagers on things like basketball games, whether or not it's going to rain, and how long it will take you to get home in this traffic.

The wages can be silly sexual things like "you have to lick peanut butter off of my nipples" or intense wagers like "you have to make me cum when we get home". You can one-up each other's wagers and set your own terms before you agree on the final bet.

To experiment with this challenge, pick a Sunday afternoon where the two of you spend the day together, taking turns setting wagers. After the Sex Bucket List is complete, you might find yourselves carry this game on well into your future.

Porn Night

Take turns picking a porn- it doesn't matter the category. Start out with some categories neither of you watch on your own like MILF or Bondage to warm up- these are categories that you can both giggle about together and maybe get some new ideas. Go in with the mindset that this is going to be an entertaining activity together...while we all know that it's impossible not to get turned on during the process. Eventually, start showing each other what you really like to watch...and see how long you can go without turning the night into your own porno.

The 10-Minute Rule

The dominant partner in this scenario sets a timer for 10 minutes. In those ten minutes, they tease their submissive partner relentlessly- nothing is off-limits.

The catch? The submissive partner is not allowed to touch the dominant partner until the timer goes off. But watch out, that timer will release a ravenous beast.

Strip Poker

Or Strip Chess. Or Strip Checkers. Or Strip Battle Ship. You can turn any game into a stripping game if you just believe in yourselves. This kind of playful spirit brings out the flirt in both of you. The tease of watching clothes slowly coming off is wonderfully torturous. And that competitive edge will add a little spice to your dynamic.

If you want to step the game up one more level, you can make a rule that whomever is naked first receives a penalty of some slutty sex act or spankings

Weird Bonus Challenge: Tarzan and Jane

Bringing animal planet to the bedroom, things are about to get rough in this male pursuit/female resistance game. Secure ropes or ties to the corners of the bed. The goal is for Tarzan to wrestle Jane into submission, getting both of her hands and legs tightly secured. Jane's job is to resist.

While this 'Tarzan and Jane' might sound rapey, with a partner that you trust, this game can be so hot. It starts out playful and funny, then all of a sudden, your inner animal is unleashed, and you end up having the best rough and angry sex.

Finished the Challenge?

You dirty kids...

But hey, you're not done yet.

Now both of you need to scan through the past 100 sexual experiences and pick your top 5 sexual experiences. Which naughty acts did you play over and over again in your head at work. Which one made you cum the hardest? Which one do you want to try again until you can perfect it?

Write them down and take turns reading them to each other, one by one.

Chapter 17: Setting the Mood

The actions leading up to the sex part is every bit as important as the sex itself. Guys, there's absolutely nothing pleasurable about simply shoving your tool in your partner and hoping she gets off when you get off. While guys have it fairly easy when it comes to sexual arousal and orgasms, girls take a little longer to heat up. This is why it's important to set the mood just right and get a girl good, wet, and ready before doing the deed. This way, you'll be able to really perform excellently in bed. That being said, here are some tips on how to get this done:

Foreplay...Duh
This seems a little obvious but unfortunately, a lot of guys don't seem to grasp the idea of foreplay properly. For most guys, foreplay is the length of time it takes to get hard enough for erection – but girls often need a longer time than that. In the later Chapters, you'll get a more detailed look on foreplay, the different erogenous parts of the body and what you can do to those parts in pursuance of foreplay.

What's important about foreplay however is to YOU TAKE YOUR TIME. This advice is mostly for the guys who want to get to the main event as quickly as possible. This is far from flattering for most women and will not lead to mutual pleasure. Hit as many erogenous zones as possible, making sure that she is very much aroused before attempting penetration. Now, some girls might be easier to arouse while others may take longer. There's no prescribed amount of minutes you'll have to devote towards foreplay – but you'll find that the more skillful you are, the faster your results.

How Do You Know She's Ready?

How do you know a girl is ready for penetration? It's a little tougher for women but most guys use lubrication as a way of finding out whether the female is ready or not. Using the fingers, males can insert it in the vagina and find out the extent of the wetness of the female. The vagina naturally releases a lubricant when the female is aroused since this helps the penis fully enter the body with as little pain as possible. There are other signs which will be discussed further later on.

Comfort and Privacy

Unless the two of you get off on having sex in less than private places, there's really nothing like comfort and privacy to get you started. This is especially true for women who can't really enjoy sex unless they're somewhere they can completely relax. For the males setting up the stage for sex – find a location that your partner is comfortable in. You'll find that this makes her very uninhibited and therefore ensures passionate response.

Striptease

A striptease is also a good way to set the stage – and this option is usually utilized by females. There's something about taking clothes off one garment at a time that gets guys wonderfully ready for sex. It works even better if the clothes themselves are sexy and layered in such a way that it provides tantalizing glimpses of the body one covering at a time.

The opposite also holds true for seduction. Removing the clothes of your partner can also be highly arousing and is considered a ritual in some countries. By removing your partner's clothes one by one, you'll be able to keep the pleasure simmering and increase the anticipation so that both become highly sensitized in time for foreplay.

Clean and Fresh

If a guy wants a girl to go down on him – a thorough bath, scrubbing all the parts that need to be scrubbed, should be performed before anything else. It's only polite and the clean smell makes women more eager to hit all those erogenous spots.

Ladies, this goes both ways. If you want a guy to pay attention to the body hotspots and linger on the foreplay, it matters very much to be clean and fresh. This is especially true if you're hoping for some oral sex. A lot of males also prefer their women to be clean-cut down under since it makes everything easier and more pleasurable to the tongue. More on that will be discussed later.

Dirty Talk

It is usually the males who love dirty talk but women also find it arousing. The concept of dirty talk is pretty blurry but for the most part, this involves being explicit about what you want or what you feel. For example, a girl might be straightforward in telling a guy that she wants his cock in her mouth or his mouth suckling her breasts. It may also involve complimenting a guy about his length or girth as he penetrates. The words 'cock', 'cunt', and 'pussy' are fairly common in dirty talk and often used in lieu of the words penis and vagina.

Another plus of dirty talk is the fact that it makes it easier for men and women to communicate about what they want in the bedroom. Does she want it harder and faster? Does she like it slow? Does he like it deep? These are information that aren't typically divulged pre-sex but can be easily provided during the throes of the act. For most, describing what you want to do or what you want done is a turn-on in itself.

Dirty talk best works with women during foreplay as men get descriptive about what they want to do for the female. Talking about how you want to suck her breasts or eat her out can be a big turn-on for women. For men, however, it's all about sensation. Talking about how good his cock feels or how big it stretches you out can boost the male ego and male the sex more pleasurable for the guy.

Bedroom Games

If you've heard of 50 Shades of Grey, you'll have a pretty good idea about bedroom games and how you can make the sex more exciting. Roleplay is a fairly common way of keeping things interesting and can offer some of the most mind-blowing sexual encounters between you and your partner. The use of toys would also be helpful. In a later Chapter, you'll find out more about sex toys and how to best utilize them to keep each other satisfied.

Porn

This is a grey area for most couples. While guys have no problem getting a hard-on while watching porn, some women will need a longer time to get aroused. However, watching porn really does help set the stage when it comes to sex, letting your partner get the message as soon as the scene starts to play.

When it comes right down to it, there are lots of things couples can do to set the mood for sex. From the vanilla to the alarming, what's really important about preludes to sex is that both partners find it arousing and are 100% consensual about the whole thing.

Chapter 18: Overcoming Sexual Inhibitions

I have dedicated a whole chapter to overcoming our sexual inhibitions because a lot of people are held back from achieving a fulfilling sexual life by sexual inhibitions they or their partners have. Most of the sexual inhibitions are brought about by being timid or bodily insecurities we may have. We all come from different backgrounds. Cultures and upbringing might dictate what we consider as taboo. Our experiences and stereotypes we have heard might also influence our sexual lives.

One of the issues that relationships experts agree hinders a full sex life are inhibitions. All over the world, people have different inhibitions that come from the subconscious mind and greatly affect our sexual behavior. Mostly negative influences form the basis of our inhibitions. Inhibitions can be said to be self-imposed restrictions. Common inhibitions that women suffer from include the good girl syndrome. Their subconscious mind is always keeping guard against doing anything that can get them labeled as a bad girl.

These activities such as masturbation, stripping, oral sex and anal sex are considered taboo. Initiating sex is also considered by some as a man's thing. A women's body can also cause inhibitions. Shape and sizes vary widely. However, mainstream media have often portrayed beautiful women as only those with a slim often unhealthy figure. All these things make a woman become self-conscious and makes her keep her guard up during sex. This limits the extent to which you can enjoy your sex life.

For men, the greatest inhibition often comes with the size of his penis. Men have been made to understand that size matters. That you cannot satisfy a woman if you have an average sized member. This is often driven by the porn industry where models with super-sized penises are displayed. Most men don't take into consideration that this is a very small fraction of the male population who have been chosen to act in this industry specifically due to this quality. Another inhibition men may have is anxiety regarding their performance in bed. The anxiety leads to poor performance and the cycle continues.

Lots of sexual inhibitions will prevent you from achieving a full sex life. Note that, sex is about exploration. Always discovering new things with our partners and reaching new heights of passion that we never had before. A full sex life involves remaining open minded about trying new things. Repeating the same things over and over again quickly becomes boring and that's when you hear couples say that they view sex as a duty or one of the chores they have to do. You never have to get to this point. To overcome sexual inhibitions you need to:

Reflect on yourself: This will involve looking inwards and identifying that which holds you back. However, this is easier said than done. Not many people are willing to look inwards; human nature is that we always tend to look at the other person when things are going as expected. Before we look at our partners we need to look at ourselves. You might have had a bad sexual experience in the past which always holds you back when it comes to fully submitting yourself to your partner. For instance women and even men who have suffered sexual abuse in the past find it difficult to fully express themselves sexually. Are your cultural and religious beliefs holding you back? Are you embarrassed to have a discussion with your partner about sex? Do you have any insecurity? Once you identify what holds you back, work on it with your partner and find the best way to overcome it. If you need assistance, seek it from a professional. Life is too short to not enjoy sex!

Come up with a plan: Once you understand your inhibitions and where they stem from, you should come up with a plan on how to overcome them. Deeply rooted issues or long held beliefs will take time to overcome. However, if you are willing and your partner supports you, it becomes even easier. You might also need professional help form a qualified individual. Insecurities we might hold might only exist in our heads. Your partner might not have a problem at all. However, you might hit a gym or enroll in a fitness program if it makes you feel better. A healthier lifestyle involving healthy diet and exercises is a good foundation for a satisfying sex life.

Communicate your fears to your partner: Communication is the only way you can work on and solve a problem especially when it comes to sex. Choosing to avoid communication only worsens the situation. However, challenging the conversation maybe, you have to speak with your partner and let them know your insecurities, fears, inhibitions, so that you can work on them. Your partner will also offer positive reinforcement every time they notice your inhibitions are holding you back. Likewise, we should aim to understand our partner's inhibitions and help them overcome them. There's not anyone person in this world that doesn't have some form of inhibition.

Understand your limits: inhibitions are not always bad. Some inhibitions are there to help us avoid physical and emotional harm. Understanding our limits and explaining them to our partners is a good way to ensure we enjoy sex while at the same time protecting ourselves. Learn your limits and explain them clearly. If something puts you off, you should tell your partner clearly. Likewise, we should learn and understand our partners' limits and respect them.

Once you cultivate this culture of trust and respect in your relationship, you are more likely to be open to new things. You will have the confidence that your partner understands your limits and will always respect them. You will then drop your guard and enjoy sex.

Chapter 19: Crazy Positions and Places/Situation Where to Have Sex (Ex Washing Machine, On the Stairs, Etc) Spicy Tips

We all give out the vibes that we desire good sex just like the oxygen that breath, in as much as we desire sex positions that will give us spine-tingling, back toe-curling, back arching, and mind-blowing orgasm but it can be frustrating if this literally happens in a split second when all we needed was a sex session that is so passionate and we can relish for a long while. Because it worth every bit to satisfy our partners sexually then we should be ready to recharge, revive and reload our naughty bits so as to keep our partners spell-bound in the bedroom which will help them last longer and always feel horny anytime they are with us.

The sure way to make partners last longer on bed is just to change the sex position repertoire. Slow and steady naughty sex positions can be of immense help here. Sex positions that will make partners take a breather and readjust their pace can be introduced while partners unleash their wild side and tap into each other animalistic urges and really blow off the sexual steam. Below are 10 tantalizing and sizzling sex positions that you can use to overwhelm your partner with intense pleasure while having it subtle and slow to have a longer sex session together.

- **The lap dance sex position**

This raunchy sex position can get any man to the clouds with intense pleasure, whether it by sucking or rubbing the tip of the cock before allowing him to penetrate, but it sure going to be shallow penetration so that both will not be over stimulated to get to orgasm very fast. The partners are sure going to give each other some orgasmic thrilling to get them going steadily before climaxing. This is one sex position that the man will relax and enjoy the stimulation from the woman even as the woman makes herself more visually appealing by pressing her boobs on his chest while giving him a massage on the scrotum. With this sex position the man sit first on a surface with his leg wide open while the woman will be on her feet backing the man, then she will gently lower yourself and grab his penis and guide it into her vagina, then grind slowly on your man, then, she can intermittently increase the intensity by bouncing her booty up and down to give him some real pleasure, she can as well bend forwards or backward to get the full length of the erected penis right inside her. At the same time the woman can look over her shoulder and make eye contact and kiss the man, she should continue with slow and subtle grinding which will enable them last longer before they both let out screaming orgasms.

- **The valedictorian sex position**

The valedictorian sex position is a very seductive sex position that can elicit overtly strong excitement for partners that uses it, this sex position involves slow grinding that will pleasure both partners and makes them go weak in the knee in response to all the naughty things they are slowly doing to their body. Like the thrills is killing them softly. Oral sex can be used with this sex position to put the partners in a euphoria that will get them to the seventh heaven. With The valedictorian sex position the woman lie on her back while your man is on top just like the missionary sex position but this time around the woman will raise his two legs up and extend them straight out to form a v shape, this will allow the cock to have a shallow contact with the vulva so as to have slow thrusting from the man so as to enable the man remain in the woman for a long time. To heighten the sensation the woman can use her hands to give the man a massage and intermittently suck the penis before directing it back to her vagina. The man can then ride the woman to stupor while the woman holds his waist as the climax together.

- **The cross sex position**

The cross sex position is a suggestive sex position to pump pleasure into the entire sensual parts of each partner's body. This sex position can make the partner's adrenaline level pump up as fast as possible, because the pleasure that will engulf them will be uncontrollable with this sex position. The penetration with this sex position will be deeper but at controllably rate and each thrust will come with its sensation that will stupefy partners and make them come with an earth-quaking screams. To achieve this the man lies on his side facing the woman, while the woman lie on her back perpendicular to the man's body with her leg draped over the side of the man's pelvis, the woman press her crotch up against the man's own and she open her legs so that the man can penetrate easily. The man penetrates from that angle moving back and forth and holding onto the woman's thighs for leverage. The woman can also respond to the motion by pushing herself closer to get each thrust as the man slowly thrusts away. While the free hands move up and down on the sensual parts of the body. The woman can let the man have a good view of her clitoris by parting her labia a bit wide to drive him sexually crazy, the woman can also work her waist to the rhythm of the man's thrust, to give him that toe-curling feelings. The woman should keep the penis tight in her throughout each thrusting still they explode in multiple orgasms.

- **The flatiron sex position**

Partners wanting to last longer during sex can't go wrong using this unique sex position. This sex position offers long lasting pleasure as the partners subtly rock themselves to unforgettable ecstasy. flatiron sex position allow the partners to take a break and reconnect again so that they will enjoyed themselves and still be sexually active for a good duration of time. A lot of couples will love this sex position, not with the position allowing the man's cock to fill up the woman's vagina and tightly glued to the vagina because of this position. This sizzling hot position enable lot of spanking and stimulation of the partners' erogenous zones that will help heighten the pleasure they will receive. Flatiron sex positions have the woman lying on her stomach on the bed in a plank position while the man straddles her. The woman raises her hips towards the man to allow for deeper penetration because the tighter the penis in the woman, the more sensation the couples will feel. So instead of the man to be fast and pounding he will go slowly but grinding deeply for good amount of sensation. The man will intermittently change from oral sex to vagina sex to give room for lasting effects. So partners that need to last longer during sex should try out this sex position and the woman shouldn't forget to lift her hip intermittently to help keep the penis in her for a long time.

- **Butterfly**

Couples that use this sex position are sure to last longer during any steamy sex session. This sex position would not just make couples last longer in bed but get the woman dripping wet and making the partners go crazy with multiple orgasms. If couples need to get mind-blowing and spine tingling pleasure then this sex position is sure to provide all of that. Butterfly sex position offers visual appeal because every inch of the body will be on display and of course this is an erotic way of evoking sexual bliss. With butterfly sex position partners are sure to be overwhelmed in ecstasy as they ride and do other naughty things to the body. The woman will lie on her back while the man stands or kneels next to the woman to enter from that angle but before penetration, foreplay can be started with the woman sitting on the man face to take oral sex and the man can be touching the woman mound to create more sexual tension. One or two sexual toys can be thrown in to the mix, this will create more frenzy and the woman body will be ready to penetrate, the woman can go back to the former position while the man penetrates her while she holds his waist for support, The woman should move her own waist with the man rhythm and let out some moans to get the man crazy. The man goes grinding in a circular form to keep the steady and slow tempo for a long-lasting effect. The woman can also give him oral sex by sucking his cock and directing the penis back to her juice dripping vagina, the man continues with the thrusting while the woman touches the man other kiss-ass erogenous zones still both of them erupt in uncontrollable orgasm.

- **The sitting sex position**

This is another sex position that will help rock couple's sexual world in no hold barred manner. This sex position is a sweet and sensual one can make couple's screw-off their head because this sex position gives a perfect intense pleasure that is unimaginable. So if you need a sex position that will help you and your partner last longer during sex, the sitting sex position is what you need to try out. It is one sex position couples might take some breaks without killing the active sexual activity going on till they both erupt in multiple orgasmic thrills that will leave them both drained. Performing this sex position start with the man sitting down upright on his butt, the woman goes down first to elongate the erection of the penis by sucking it, then she slowly lower herself on the man by sitting and facing him. The man grabs the woman's breast and sucks it while his hand is playing with the woman clit to swell it up. Thereafter, the woman uses her hand to guide the man's penis into her vagina but can first press the cock against her clit to elicit pleasure and really get wet. She then let the penis in. The woman can wrap her legs around the man's back and put her arms around the man's neck for leverage. To add more sensation and intimacy the hands at the back can be used for a massage. The woman can move up and down or grind her hips in tantalizing circles and from there they can both synchronize moving forth and back in a rhythm. They both can steadily increase the sexual tempo thrusting in that position till they both erupt in uncontrollable ecstasy.

- **The sidewinder sex position**

The sidewinder sex position is one sex position that partners and couples can use to mesmerize one another in the bedroom. It's one sex position that can give couples the orgasmic thrills they really needs as well as helping them last longer in bed. This sex position enable partners to once in a while stop and make out with some kisses and dry humping before slowing thrusting away to make them last longer. If you are thinking of a tantalizing sex position you will relish with your partner while staying with one another a bit longer, then checking out the sidewinder sex position will be your best option. It will surely make both partners go gaga in sexual excitement. Performing the sidewinder sex position needs both partners laying down and facing each other on the sides. The woman will lift her upper leg so that the man would penetrate from that angle. Then the woman wrap her leg tightly around the man's own legs so that the man can use her muscles and friction to thrust strongly, The woman can keep her legs close together to give the man an extra snug fit for more powerful stimulation. A blowjob can be given to the man by the woman, then she can use her hands to massage his inner thighs, lick his balls then she can tease his penis before sliding it into her mouth. To get the enjoyment of rear entry and the naughty thrills of this sex position but without overly intense stimulation that will birth lesser sex position, the man will penetrate the woman from the rear end as described above position and give some slow thrusting though deeply for longer session and also build orgasmic thrills till they explode in ecstasy that is unimaginable and climax afterwards.

- **Waterfall sex position**

Waterfall sex position is an erotic sex position that partners that needs longer sex session should experiment with, because it one sex position that partners will have a jolly ride pleasuring one another. This sex position gives partners a head rush that is memorable, the sensation that erupts from this sex position during the sex session is heavenly, and you can't go wrong using this sex position if you need a sex position that will enable you to last longer with your partner while having real hot sex session. This is one sex position that partners can use to mesmerize one another in the bedroom. With this sex position the man lay on his back on the bed with his shoulders and head hanging down on the floor, then the woman goes on top and then start with foreplay, she can start with the sexy mouth moves to give the man an early arousal by kissing his ears, his neck, his thigh, his stomach and using her hands to give him a massage. She can arouse further by giving him oral sex through licking his balls, sucking his nipples and cock. She can then lower herself slowly on his cock and start thrusting subtly in circles to inhibit quick ejaculation intermittently she let the penis press on her clit to send sexual waves to their body. The woman can go further to squeeze the muscles of your vulva a bit to hold the penis tightly and then increase the tempo of the sensation by riding hard a bit. She can let her booty bounce back and forth before him for more visual appeal and to induce the man to unconsciously moan and scream in ecstasy. She can take a break for more caresses and kisses before riding harder this time to climax.

- **Sofa surprise position**

This is a sex position that one can perform anywhere on the bed, in the bathtub, the kitchen etc so don't be deceived by the name because it isn't only restricted to your sofa. This is almost like the Asian cowgirl sex position where the woman is on top of the man which both partners enjoy a lot. So if partners want a long lasting steaming sex session with earth quaking orgasm then trying out this sex position will be their pleasure. The man sits on a sofa or anything else and the woman squat down on the man from a standing position facing the man so that man would enter her from that angle, the woman will need to be flexible here since she will be squatting far low, then the man can stimulate the woman and get her really wet before penetrating through this angle. The woman can lift her butt a bit so that the man can penetrate the wet pussy conveniently, penetrating deep so that the penis can fill her up, if she is tired of squatting, let her sit on the man's laps and grind on it by pushing her hips forwards and backwards over him. The man can elicit more pleasure by spanking the woman's booty and tingling her nipples. The man can take over with the shallow thrusting which will help keep the session for a long time before orgasm.

- **Eyes to the sky sex position**

An eye to the sky sex position is one position that gets partners screaming and moaning to the clouds. You can't get it wrong with this naughty sex position if you are really trying to pleasure yourself and also last longer in bed. This sex position will always get couples horny any time they remembers how hot and sizzling it will be when they both get down. So if you are looking for subtle but hot sex position that will give you and your partner intense pleasure and enable you both to last longer too then try out this very juicy sex position. You can start off this tantalizing sex position having the man lie on his back while the woman assume the position on top of the man. The woman can give the man a hand job to get his erection strong enough and the woman should be well lubricated too or the man can use foreplay to get the woman dripping with juice, the woman can use her hand to steady herself on the bed while using the other hand to keep the base of your penis steady as she lower herself on the cock, she then places her back on his chest and they both face the ceiling. Then she start grinding or rocking the man, with this position since it's harder for the man to go deep, he'll last way longer and the drilling will last long so that they get all the sexual pleasure as expected before climaxing.

Chapter 20: Secret to lasting longer

Kama Sutra says that your woman must arrive at the climax, before you do; for which she might need prolonged stimulation, through sensuous kissing, petting, caressing, licking, and biting as well as oral sex. You have to prevent early ejaculation by controlling and delaying the excitement and excessive stimulation. Techniques of breathing control as well as mind control too can be helpful.

Kama Sutra focuses on how you should arouse and stimulate your princess at all of her erogenous zones, with a lot of patience and delay tactfully the actual penetration, so that both of you can have prolonged enjoyment culminating in simultaneous climaxing.

In case of a smaller diameter lingam (penis), the sex position chosen should be such that your princess should be able to squeeze her thighs together, in order to control size of yoni opening. She should also learn the technique of vagina muscle contraction, combined with hip rotation, to be able to climax early and delay male ejaculation by holding male organ static for a while.

Kama sutra prescribes certain preferred sex positions, which help you to last longer, by reducing the sensitivity of your erect penis and increasing your ability to ensure ejaculatory control.

A. The goat - tree position, which is similar to the cowgirl posture. You should be seated on a chair and your princess would be seated on your thighs facing you. She moves her hips, and thus controls the movements of your penis, and ensures a delay in build-up of your climax, to synchronize with her own orgasm.

B. Mandarin Duck is similar to spoon posture (side to side) posture. While your princess is resting on her side, you penetrate her vaginal opening from behind. This position allows her to climax early while you can exercise more control on reaching the climax, due to better ejaculatory control. Her thighs remain tightly closed, giving excess stimulation to her while controlling your strokes moderately.

C. Woman on top positions is generally known to delay your climax, so that both could climax together.

D. Positions which increases the passion in men, such as rear entry positions (Shvanaka or doggy posture, Dhenuka or Cow positions could lead to early ejaculation, if the arousal is not moderated by suitable techniques.

E. Rolling over and using a modified posture during the midsession, could help men to delay the ejaculation.

F. Other ideas and tricks of delaying your ejaculation:

experimenting with variants of the postures that stimulate women,

- And___exploring and adopting different penetration angles, which causes female orgasm more rapidly.

G. Some yoga postures and abdominal workouts can cure the problem of early male ejaculation. Pranayama, meditation and certain deep breathing methods can improve the muscles and nerves, which cause premature ejaculation.

Factors aggravating the problem include

•Mental anxiety due to some other reason,

•Lack of privacy during sex,

•Guilty feeling for certain relationships, in subconscious mind,

•Fear of being caught during sex act and

• Risk of unwanted pregnancy can also result in premature ejaculation.

H. the Kama sutra author advices use of animal and herbal based nutrients for improving sexual performance. For men it suggests

"…. try boiled testicles of goat or ram, with milk as well as sugar.

…try the boiled eggs of sparrow, boiled in milk, rice, mixed with ghee and honey.

…try juice of fenner plant, mixed with liquorice, ghee, and honey-sugar."

OtherSecret tips on bedroom performance and lasting longer:

1. The pause-squeeze

The "pause-squeeze" is one of those scientific techniques/methods for men for preventing early climax. When you're about to climax, tell your partner; withdraw from vagina, she can squeezethe "joining point" part of the penis. It is a point where head of the penis is joining the shaft. She must squeeze the point for several seconds, till your urge to climax subsides.

Now you must wait for 30-40 seconds before resuming pelvic strokes or foreplay.

Within the vagina also she can control and reduce the sensation of ejaculation, by relaxing her internal muscle and opening her thighs wider to reduce tightness

Other points on the penis to be squeezed:

base of the shaft,

underside of the head; and

Points between base of the scrotum and the anal opening.

2 practice squeeze pause during hand job

If you practice squeeze-pause during hand job, habitually you can control early ejaculation and last longer.

Couples generally confirm that they stay longer, if they masturbate some time before a love making session. Women prefer toy sex too, to have early orgasm. Women confess that they have quality orgasm when they make use of sex toys for stimulation, though they prefer the arousal through the tongue of the partner regularly. Oral sex is given by women to arouse men and confirm message of love.

3 postpone penetrating

If you postpone the penetration, you spend time in foreplay and oral sex. It takes 15 to 20 minutes for a woman to climax. Men last nearly 3 to 5 minutes after they penetrate.

4. Counseling

Professional Counseling can help you control and overcome performance anxiety, guilt and psychologically boost your confidence. If you are lasting for less than 3 minutes, you may require expert medical advice.

5 life style and herbal solutions

Have a balanced diet with a variety of fruits and vegetables. Banana, Indian gooseberry (Alma), beet-root, strawberries are some of the foods you may want to add to your diet.

A <u>popular fruit to prevent premature ejaculation has been blueberry.</u> It has package of nutrients that relax your pelvic blood vessels, thus improving the blood flow to your penis. This will help you to last longer. Consuming blueberries may cure premature ejaculation, as they contain dopamine, which is the "feel good" hormone, which regulates flow of semen during onset of the ejaculation.

Other popular herbal remedies used include:

1 nutmeg (Jaiphal)

2 asparagus adsendens

3 Gokshura (Tribulus Terrestris)

4 Garlic

5 Shilajit

6 Asva gandha or Indian ginseng found useful for male rejuvenation

7 Shatavari or asparagus racemousus (for females)

(Reduce alcohol and stop smoking. Quitting alcohol may be difficult, but may boost your chances of staying longer on long term basis.)

Yoga postures such as Bhujangasan (cobra pose) and Paschimotthanasana help flow of oxygen and blood to the genitals. Strengthen the abdominal muscles by yoga and Pranayama. (Practice deep breathing every day on an empty stomach for ten minutes).

8 practice squeeze-stop-release while urinating:

While urinating, use a squeeze- stop (Pause) - release technique. Use fifteen interruptions, each of ten seconds, while you urinate for ten seconds in between and stop again. This may be practiced thrice a day.

By interrupting urine flow, you will be exercising your pubococcygeus muscle (PC muscle); these muscles are located all over from urinary sphincter to anus. By squeezing PC muscle, you improve blood flow to penis, and you train yourself how to habitually delay ejaculation.

9 medicated condoms, Lidocain and maiden overs

Stimulation on penis head can be reduced by use of medicated condoms. Changing angle of strokes, grinding of hips in place of too and fro movement, can reduce the sensation, thus helping you stay on.

Lidocaine is a chemical injected by the dentists to reduce pain in gums. Condoms linedwith this drug Lidocaine are now available, but they need doctor's prescription. (On the other hand, a higher dosage of Lidocaine layer on the condom inner surface, may not allow erection at all.)

Initial maiden overs

Men normally do not last longer during the initial few maiden-overs. But this should not worry them. Having sex with the right females in better settings, with minimum outside interference could enhance their sexual performance subsequently.

Before the climax begins, during the intercourse, some groups of nerves, called Krause finger corpuscles, send some signals from the penis to control centers in the brain that control semen flow and ejaculation. If dopamine levels are high in the blood flow due to feeling of guilt or fear, control centers in the brain, send a urgent signal to the muscles in penis, to throw semen out quickly. Keeping the mind under control is important to reduce guilt and fear. This can be done by adopting yoga and meditation.

Postures with women on top, or alternating between men on top and woman on top, after initial penetration, can enable the male partner to stay longer.

Changing postures from rear penetration position to woman on top position can also help them to stay longer.

7to nine

Experts suggest 7 to9 technique, which means 7 superfast in-out thrusts followed by 9 slower in-out strokes. You should also use this in combination of hip rotations. These require mental alertness as well.

Chapter 21: Adventurous Positions

This chapter is full of sex positions that can help you show your wild side. In certain cases, you just have to let go and make love to your partner with reckless abandon. With these positions, you can forget about foreplay rituals and just satisfy your carnal needs.

The Circle

This position allows the couple to take submissive and dominant roles. The woman lies on her back and assumes a knotted position. The man, on the other hand, will position himself above her and restrict her movements. Many couples think of this sex position as extremely arousing.

The steps:

1. The female must lie on the bed and spread her legs.
2. The man will kneel before his partner and stroke her thighs.
3. He has to push her knees towards her breasts. Meanwhile, he must shower her thighs with passionate kisses.
4. The man must hold her feet and cross her calves.

5. Then, he will kneel over his partner and slide his penis into her. In the final position, the woman's legs are crossed and are pinned against her breasts.

Increasing the Intensity:

- The woman may rake her fingernails on the man's chest. This action adds animalistic elements to the position.
- The man may secure his position by pinning the woman's feet between his stomach and legs.
- Before crossing the woman's calves, he may position the woman's legs according to his preferences.

The Fourth Position

In this sex position, the man has complete access to the front section of the woman's body. That means he can kiss and caress the woman's hot spots (e.g. neck, nipples, clitoris, etc.).

The steps:

1. The man has to kneel and assume a sitting position.

2. The woman will face the man and climb onto his body. She must wrap her arms around her partner's neck and press her body against his.
3. He will slide his penis into the woman and lower her onto the bed. Meanwhile, she should maintain the position by crossing her feet behind the man.
4. Slowly, she must raise her legs and rest them on the man's shoulders. The woman should move her legs one at a time.

Increasing the Intensity:

- He may improve the position's stability by holding the woman's hips. This tip becomes important while he goes in and out of her.
- The woman may lean back and expose her body to her lover.

The Intact Position

This position allows lovers to have compact and raunchy sex. It offers deep penetration, a shade of dominance, and bonus adventure.

The steps:

1. The woman will lie on her back and raise her legs.

2. The man will part her legs, climb on top of her, and penetrate her. He should support his body using his knees and hands.
3. Next, he should take a kneeling position.
4. The woman will bend her knees and draw them to her chest. This posture allows the man to penetrate the woman deeply.
5. He must lean forward so that his body is pressing against the woman's knees.

Increasing the Intensity:

- The woman may use nipple clamps to add more kinkiness to the position.
- The man may hold the woman's hair while he penetrates her. Some women enjoy tingling sensations on their scalp during sex.
- He may move the woman's butt in order to find an ideal penetration angle. This trick ensures that the man can thrust smoothly and easily.

The Rising Posture

Even though this position restricts the couple's movements, it has an excellent rating in terms of erotic tension. Here, the couple will face each other, while the woman's legs are stopping the man from getting close to her. Sex gurus claim that this is the ideal position for giving precoital orgasm to the woman.

The steps:

1. The woman will lie on her back. Then, she will pull her knees towards her breasts.
2. The man must sit on the bed and spread his legs.
3. The woman needs to place her feet on his stomach. The man, meanwhile, will penetrate her.
4. She will move her feet up to the man's chest.

Increasing the Intensity:

- The man may hold the woman's feet while he penetrates her. Here, he may either squeeze the woman's feet together or spread them apart.
- She may increase the attractiveness of her legs by wearing a garter belt and a pair of stockings.

Flying Seagulls

This position will help you satisfy all of your sexual needs. It doesn't require high-levels of fitness and flexibility. Additionally, if the man is taller than the woman, the penetration angle will produce amazing sensations. This sex position also allows you to use your hands extensively.

The steps:

1. The woman will sit on the edge of the bed. The man will kneel before her.
2. The couple will kiss each other. The woman will spread her legs, wrap them around the man's waist, and plant her feet steadily on the floor. Then, the man will penetrate his partner.
3. The woman will allow her body to fall on the bed. Then, she will relax her legs and savor the man's efforts.

Increasing the Intensity:

- The man may caress the body of his partner. Here, he can begin from her breasts down to her butt.
- He may kneel in an upright position. This posture will help him in getting an excellent penetration angle.
- The woman may help her partner in getting a deeper penetration. She may place her feet on the man's butt and drop her knees onto the bed.

The Raised Feet Position

This interesting variant of the man-on-top position has 9 sub-variants in the Kama Sutra book. Thus, even the ancient sex gurus believe in the effectiveness of this sex position.

The steps:

1. The woman will lie on her back and spread her legs. She will open herself to the man by pulling her knees toward her chest.
2. The man will kneel before the woman and spread his legs.
3. Once the man has penetrated her, the woman will rest her feet on the man's shoulders. Sex gurus use the term "Level Feet Position" when referring to this posture.
4. She will slide her feet along the man's body, slowly and sensually. The woman must rest her feet on the waist of her partner.
5. The man will bend forward above his partner.

Increasing the Intensity:

- The man should vary the depth of his thrusts. This way, the woman will experience different kinds of sensations.
- He can give her more pleasure by pressing her nipples gently.

- The woman can take an active role in this position. She may sit up, grab the man around his waist, and move against him.
- She can improve the level of penetration by tightening the grip of her legs around the man's waist.

Chapter 22: Additional Tips For Better Sex

Sex is a composition of various movements, erogenous zones, techniques, and sensations so be assured that there are always ways to make things more amazing in the bedroom. Here are some tips that can help guys and girls get the most out of each coupling.

Take Your Time

The common issue for most men with sex is that they take things too fast, failing to provide women with sufficient time to really get things in gear. Hence, she's not properly aroused and therefore unlikely to reach orgasm.

Give proper attention to the prelude or the foreplay, not just through the stimulation of the erogenous zones but also by making her comfortable and mentally ready. It is often said that the biggest and most powerful erogenous zone is the brain – which is why the Kama Sutra extensively talks about courtship and how to make the woman receptive to the advances of the male.

The Use of Sounds

Moans and other sounds coming from the female are highly arousing for many males and shows that the female is leisurely enjoying the situation. Hence, females who want to increase the satisfaction for their male partner should be vocal about the sensations they are feeling and the pleasure of the sexual act. Additional caresses, pinching, sucking, and licking aren't exclusively done by males. Women will find that performing additional tasks during sex, particularly to the erogenous zones of the male will enhance his satisfaction.

It has also been proven that men are very visual when it comes to sex. Hence, a large number of them enjoy watching the female pleasure herself during sex, either by touching her breasts or playing with the clitoris.

Alternate

The Kama Sutra talks about the need to change pace, actions, and intensity during the sexual act. The fact is that there is no specific formula for the perfect sex. Different people have different methods of enjoying the act and may require different methods for stimulation. While others are perfectly happy with the typical foreplay, others may like it better to have their lovers wearing leather or performing some service. The same is true with kissing, touching, licking, biting, and other actions. Alternating from soft to hard, fast to slow, and then vice versa can keep the passion and pleasure going, ensuring the both parties remain in the throes of sexual intensity.

You'll find that there's also no specified time length for sex. While women generally need lots of foreplay, there are situations when she is quickly and properly aroused so that there's nothing left to do but penetrate and thrust. Other times, you'd like it slow and lingering so that both parties can truly enjoy the moment. The differences and the failure to predict how the sex will occur is part of the excitement.

Talk About It

Talking about sex – whether before or after – is usually a good idea. For some couples, the conversation is done during sex. We're not talking about the 'emotional' stuff here but rather, a talk about what gets you satisfied and what doesn't. This is important because although observing the reaction of your lover is a good starting point, it doesn't always provide a clear picture of how satisfactory the sex life happens to be.

Couples are encouraged to talk about what gets them off and what sexual acts they do NOT like in the bedroom. Only through this can you perfect the sex and _{really} get satisfaction into the bargain. Remember: every person is different so you'll have to adjust your actions depending on the person you're with.

Mirrors, Videos, and Locations

You can also further boost sexual pleasure by strategically placing mirrors in different parts of the bedroom or house so that you can watch yourself having sex. This is a big turn on for guys and actually provides a whole new dimension to the sexual union. The recording of the sex can also be terribly exciting although of course, you'll have to take careful steps to ensure that no one else views the act, especially if you have no intention of becoming a porn star.

Choosing different locations in the house to have sex in also kicks up the excitement a notch. For the most part, different locations in the house make it possible for couples to be inventive with the sexual positioning. For example, wall sex is best done in the shower while table sex can be done in the dining room. At the very least, sex in different locations of the house gives couples the chance to embed a memory into the specific location, allowing them to have something pleasant to remember each time they use the facilities.

Conclusion

As you embark on your voyage toward greater intimacy and mutual awareness, you can practice positions of nurturing that will help you to restore and harmonize your energies after a fight or disagreement. And if you still don't feel comfortable doing these with your partner, practice on your own, in front of a mirror.

Choose a quiet place. Sit in a comfortable position, with you and your partner facing each other. Preferably, you are on cushions on the floor, sitting cross-legged and face-to-face, as close to each other as possible. You may sit on chairs with a straight back so you sit up straight. Relax and breathe into your belly.

Look at your partner. Your eyes should be soft and inviting. You don't have to smile or look fascinated — just relax, breathe, and allow yourself to open up to the moment. Stay together in this way for about five minutes.

Next, each of you should place your right hand on your partner's heart and your left hand over your partner's arm, on your own heart. The palms of your hands should be flat so that they are touching your partner and yourself completely. Breathe and eye gaze. Relax into the feeling of complete surrender. Stay present with your partner and focus your awareness on only the two of you.

Eye gazing during the act of sex is a very powerful experience. We are open and vulnerable at that time. Once you are more comfortable with doing it, see if you can look into your lover's eyes while you orgasm. This may be more difficult — you're probably conditioned to go inside, thinking you'll feel the experience more. In truth, you may actually be able to expand the orgasmic feelings more when you are fully connected to your partner through your eyes.

This is an excellent exercise to clear negative energy that can arise from everyday fights and disagreements. Lie on your side with your partner, with one of you in front of the other, like spoons in a drawer. If you are in back, place your top arm over your partner and hold your hand to her heart. If you are in front, have your partner place her hand on your heart. Relax and breathe together. Do this for at least five minutes.

After a few minutes, you can also try some slow, gentle undulating together. One of you starts and begins to rock from the hips. Cradle your partner in your arms and hold firmly. This is a good tool for getting in sync or harmonizing.

www.ingramcontent.com/pod-product-compliance
Lightning Source LLC
Chambersburg PA
CBHW070903080526
44589CB00013B/1167